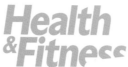

YOGA

A beginner's guide

Words and yoga instruction **Eve Boggenpoel**
Editor **Mary Comber**
Art editor **Kelly Flood**
Chief sub-editor **Sheila Reid**

Photography **Danny Bird @ Tapestry**
Hair & make-up **Nathalie Fournier @ Artistic Licence**
Model **Kim Hartwell @ WModels**
Retouching (inside) **Colin Beagley**

Publisher **Steven O'Hara**
Publishing Director **Dan Savage**
Marketing Manager **Charlotte Park**
Commercial Director **Nigel Hole**

Printed by **William Gibbons and Sons, Wolverhampton**

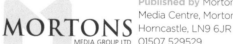

Published by Mortons Media Group Ltd,
Media Centre, Morton Way,
Horncastle, LN9 6JR
01507 529529

MAGBOOK

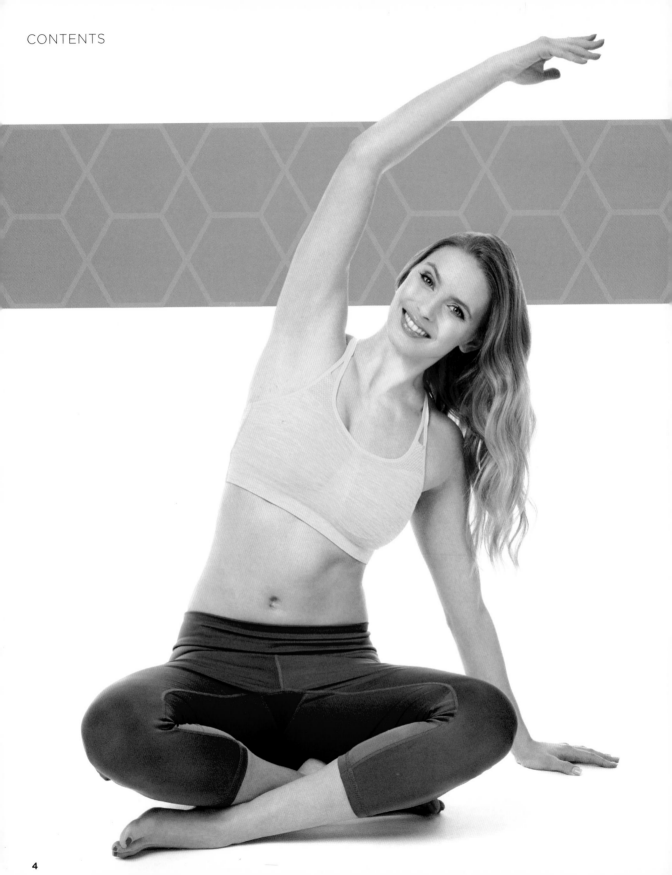

Contents

"Today is your opportunity to make your tomorrow better"

Dalai Lama

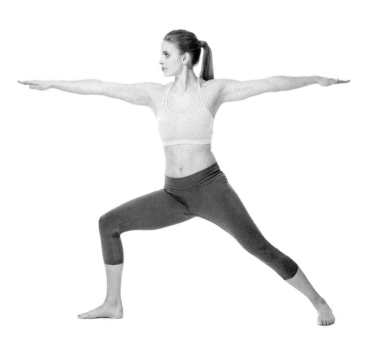

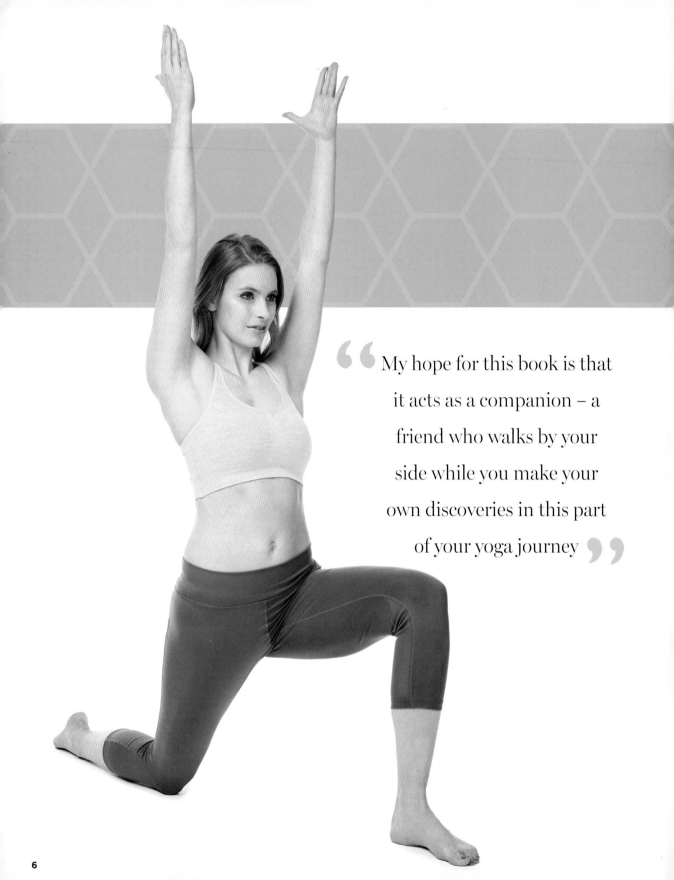

"My hope for this book is that it acts as a companion – a friend who walks by your side while you make your own discoveries in this part of your yoga journey"

Welcome...

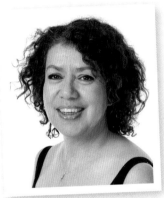

I first encountered yoga many years ago, long before the age of DVDS, streaming apps and YouTube channels.

In fact, my first forays into yoga began by scouring the hushed isles of my local library looking for any book I could find to satisfy my hunger for this enticing new form of exercise I'd heard about. Tucked away in my tiny teenager's bedroom, in between reading pony manuals and ballet novels, I would pour over the books and try to glean as much information as I could.

While learning yoga from a book is not a replacement for hands-on advice from a teacher standing next to you, the beauty of a book is that you can take your time reading the advice, studying the images and gleaning useful tips from someone who has travelled this pathway before you, so that it slowly seeps into your being and becomes part of who you are becoming.

From my early days as a yoga student, to designing my first beginner's course and later planning lessons for my own students, I discovered a love of creating sequences and planning lessons that take you on a journey – whether that's a six-week course which supports a complete beginner into becoming a level one student, or a single class that somehow transforms a stressed individual to a calmer, more centred one.

My hope for this book is that it acts as a companion – a friend that walks by your side you while you make your own discoveries in this part of your yoga journey. You may encounter many fellow travellers, both teachers and students, but if you are honest with yourself, stay true to yourself and always follow your heart, you won't go far wrong.

ABOUT THE AUTHOR

Eve Boggenpoel has been practising yoga and meditation for 25 years. Self-taught initially, her formal yoga journey began with a German Iyengar teacher when she learnt to value the significance of good alignment, and went on to include vinyasa and yin styles with inspirational teachers Shiva Rea, Sarah Powers and Simon Low.

Eve is a qualified homeopath and health journalist, and author of several books, including *Yoga Calm, 10-Minute Mindfulness, Yoga Cures* and *10-Minute AM/PM Yoga.* In *Yoga A Beginner's Guide,* Eve brings together her in-depth knowledge of yoga to create an easy-to-use guide to enhance your wellbeing in everyday life.

Eve
Eve Boggenpoel,
Author *Yoga A Beginner's Guide*

For Tom - again and always

Your 6-week
YOGA COURSE

Before you start your beginner's yoga course, read these
guidelines to find your way around the book

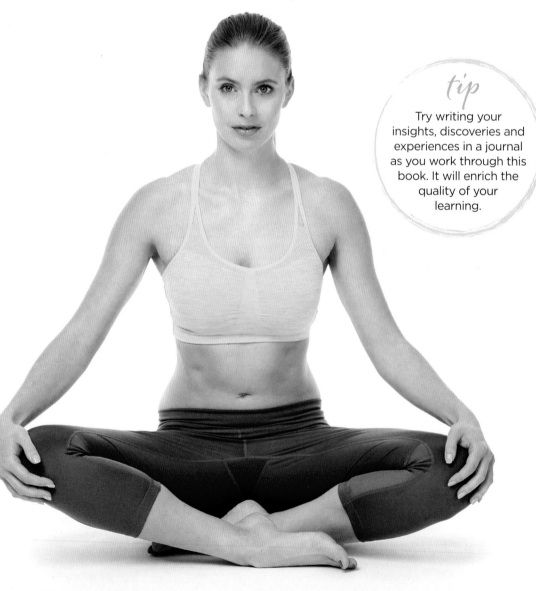

tip

Try writing your
insights, discoveries and
experiences in a journal
as you work through this
book. It will enrich the
quality of your
learning.

To learn anything well, it's important to start at the beginning, and yoga is no exception. In this book you'll find a six-week course that will guide you through the foundations of yoga and teach you the key poses and sequences you need to build up a daily yoga practice.

Take your time to read The Basics section (p10) and pose guides before you get on your mat, to give yourself the best possible start. The step-by-step instructions will ensure that you stay safe and they'll introduce you to important principles that you'll need to practise many poses. Some of these foundations, such as how to place your feet or how to breathe, are repeated several times throughout the course, so things you find challenging in Week One will become second nature by Weeks Two and Three.

While the chapters in this book are divided into six weeks, you may prefer to spend more than a week on each stage. Everyone is individual, so allow yourself to learn at a pace that suits you, and only move on to the next chapter when you feel ready. On the other hand, you may enjoy a week so much or find that it is so suited to your circumstances that you simply wish to repeat it.

One of the goals of yoga is to know and care for yourself better, so begin now and follow your inner guide as you learn.

> **Everyone is individual, so allow yourself to learn at a pace that suits you**

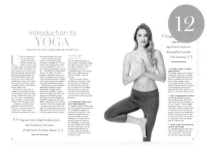

About yoga
Learn the history of yoga and the many styles of yoga that exist. Find the best type to suit you and discover the various benefits it brings.

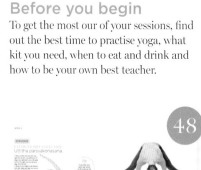

Before you begin
To get the most our of your sessions, find out the best time to practise yoga, what kit you need, when to eat and drink and how to be your own best teacher.

Finding inspiration
Now you've learnt the basics, it's time to get started! Each week we'll offer a few words of inspiration to guide you on your yoga path. Turn to them whenever you need to tune into a yogic frame of mind.

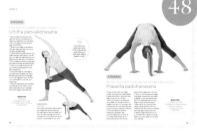

Your how-to guides
This is where you'll learn the new poses you need for the current week's lesson. Read the instructions carefully and practise the pose before you complete the class.

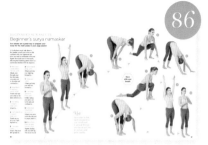

Putting it all together
At the end of each chapter, the one-hour yoga class lets you put everything you've learnt into practice. The lesson begins with a key pose that highlights that week's main principles.

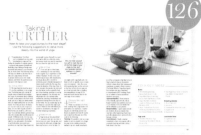

The next step
In this section discover new ways to practise yoga, learn how to spot a good teacher and discover the best resources to take your yoga journey to the next level.

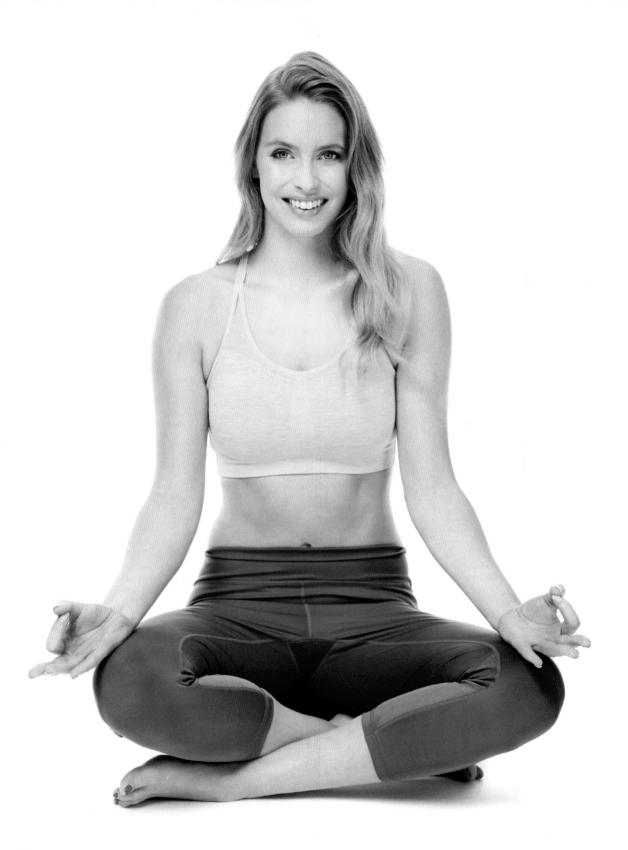

The basics

Welcome to the start of your **yoga** journey. Here you'll discover the many **benefits** of yoga and find a style that suits your **goals**. You'll also learn everything you need to get started – from essential kit to the best time **to practise**, the importance of warming up your body and how to create the ideal space for your yoga sessions.

Introduction to
YOGA

Discover the many ways yoga can benefit you

Until you've experienced it for yourself it's hard to really understand the difference a regular yoga practice can make to your life. People speak of improved flexibility, increased strength, better balance and greater stamina, but the benefits go far beyond the physical. Along with better sleep, deeper relaxation, greater focus and increased feelings of calm, yoga can give you a sense of purpose and belonging that is hard to beat. Perhaps these words from Rolf Gates, author of *Meditations from the Mat* (Bantam, £12.90) explain it best.

'When I hear the word yoga I see sunlight coming through the window of a sacred space. I hear autumn leaves moving to a gentle breeze under a blue sky. I feel a summer lake tickling my ankles, its surface a miraculous glass reflection of the mountains around it.

'I remember a room full of people taking the first deep breath they've had all day. I experience a joy too big to name. This is what it means to understand yoga, finding one's home - in this breath, this body, this moment.'

To get the most from your yoga practice, it's worth understanding something of its background. The word yoga has many meanings, but one that everyone understands is 'to yoke' or 'to unite'. While some yogis believe we are all one – meaning there is nothing separate that has to be 'united' – the idea of bringing our mind, body and spirit into balance, and being in harmony with our environment and community, inevitably creates a sense of peace and compassion most people understand and long for.

With its roots in an Indian philosophy called Vedanta, the physical yoga we practise today was largely used as a preparation for meditation to achieve those aims. Brought to the West by BSK Iyengar (who developed the Iyengar style of yoga, p12) and SK Pattabhi Jois (the father of astanga yoga, p15), many different yoga styles have since developed (see p14-15), but the focus remains similar – a practice that can help you find inner calm, outer strength and the means to live a life more in tune with your true self. It's no wonder yoga has become so popular.

Find the right yoga for you

With its increasing popularity, new forms of yoga are continually emerging, from partner yoga (yoga in pairs) and acro yoga (a combination of yoga and acrobatics), arial yoga (in a yoga trapeze/sling) to more unusual styles, such as laughter yoga, beer yoga and even doga – yoga with your dog.

There will be plenty of time to specialise as your experience of yoga grows, but for now, the following list of the main types of yoga will give you an idea of what is available. Ask yourself what you most want to achieve from your practice then, when you're ready to take your yoga to the next level, choose the appropriate style for you.

● I'm interested in static poses and in-depth alignment

Try: Iyengar Developed by BSK Iyengar, this style of yoga gives precise attention to correct alignment, giving you a good basis for all yoga styles. It was Iyengar who popularised the use of props such as blocks and straps, enabling you to experience the full benefits of a pose even before you have full flexibility. You often hold the poses for longer periods of time than other styles of yoga – good for building strength, flexibility and awareness. Iyengar also developed set sequences to help ease stress and heal physical illness.

Yoga can reduce high blood pressure,

bad cholesterol and stress,

all risk factors for heart disease

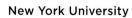

New York University

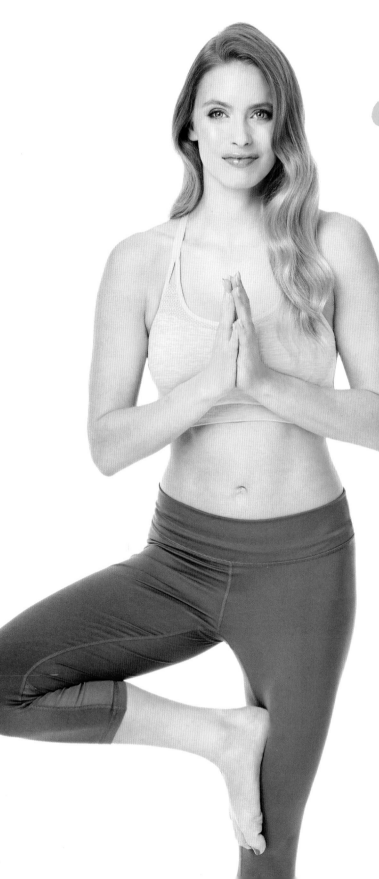

> **Eight weeks of daily yoga practice significantly improves sleep quality in people with insomnia**
>
> **Harvard University**

● **I'd prefer to follow a flowing yoga sequence**

Try: **Vinyasa** Vinyasa means 'arranged in a special way', so the poses in a vinyasa class will be carefully sequenced so that they flow seamlessly from one into the other to bring a meditative quality to your practice. Vinyasa is also used to describe a sequence of poses (Low plank, Upward-facing dog and Downward-facing dog) that may be repeated in a sun salute or at other points during the class.

● **I want a tough physical workout**

Try: **Hot yoga** Originally associated with Bikram yoga, many studios offer classes where the rooms are heated to 30 or even 50 degrees C. While the higher temperatures cause you to sweat more, said to help you release unwanted toxins, it's important not to over do it at a hot yoga class. You'll feel more flexible due to the heat, but that could leave you open to a greater risk of injury. Other forms of hot yoga include Forrest yoga, Baptiste yoga and corepower yoga.

● **I'd like to learn more about the spiritual side of yoga**

Try: **Sivananda** Sivananda classes often begin with Sun salutations then move on to 12 main poses – most of which are in this book. Along with postures,

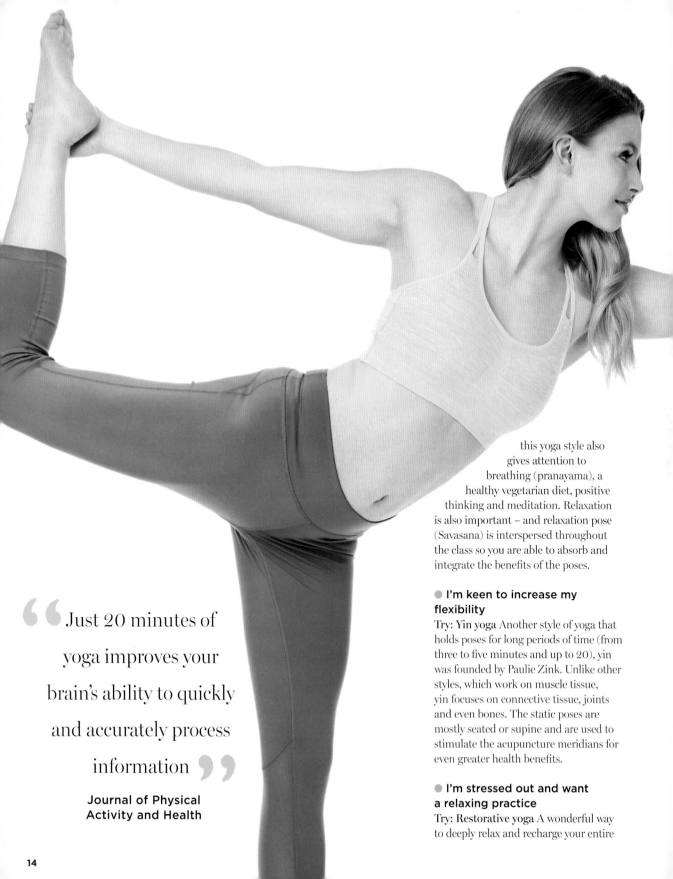

this yoga style also gives attention to breathing (pranayama), a healthy vegetarian diet, positive thinking and meditation. Relaxation is also important – and relaxation pose (Savasana) is interspersed throughout the class so you are able to absorb and integrate the benefits of the poses.

● I'm keen to increase my flexibility

Try: **Yin yoga** Another style of yoga that holds poses for long periods of time (from three to five minutes and up to 20), yin was founded by Paulie Zink. Unlike other styles, which work on muscle tissue, yin focuses on connective tissue, joints and even bones. The static poses are mostly seated or supine and are used to stimulate the acupuncture meridians for even greater health benefits.

● I'm stressed out and want a relaxing practice

Try: **Restorative yoga** A wonderful way to deeply relax and recharge your entire

> " Just 20 minutes of yoga improves your brain's ability to quickly and accurately process information "
>
> **Journal of Physical Activity and Health**

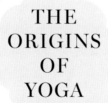

THE ORIGINS OF YOGA

The first book to describe the practice of yoga was written about 2,000 years ago. Called the *Yoga Sutras*, the author, an Indian sage known as Patanjali, describes yoga as a practice for calming the fluctuations of the mind. Still a useful way to describe yoga today, Patanjali described eight practices – the limbs of yoga – to help people achieve just that. The poses we practise today – known as asanas – are just one of these limbs. While you don't need to be a dedicated yogi to practise them, they give a valuable insight into the breadth of yoga. The eight limbs include:

system, restorative yoga classes only include four or five poses. You'll mostly be lying on your mat, using an array of bolsters, blocks, straps and blankets to support your body in such a way that your muscles can completely relax while still gently stretching. Restorative yoga also balances your nervous system, boosts immunity and improves your body's capacity to heal.

● I'd like a set sequence I can do on a regular basis

Try: Ashtanga Ashtanga yoga is divided into six series, although most people focus on series one and two. There are around 50 postures in total, along with Sun salutations, and every time you practise, you repeat the poses in a set order. You'll work hard, sweating profusely and detoxifing your muscles and organs. The result? Improved circulation, a light and strong body, and a calm mind.

● I like to work at my own pace

Try: Mysore A style of self-practice in the ashtanga tradition, Mysore sessions usually take place early in the morning and last two to three hours – although you can drop in for as long or as little as suits you. There's no formal group instruction – you work at your own pace, and the teacher gives you guidance individually. Beginners are taught a Sun salutation and additional poses are offered as you become ready.

Yamas These are five moral restrains for living, involving not harming anything including ourselves; being truthful; not stealing; exercising moderation; and not being greedy.

Niyamas The second limb of yoga is five precepts for healthy living: cleanliness, contentment, discipline, study and contemplation.

Asana The physical poses we are familiar with today, they were originally designed to prepare the body for meditation.

Pranayama Breathing exercises that can energise or calm your mind, balance your body, purify your system and clear blocked energy.

Pratyahara This refers to practices where you withdraw your senses, essentially

bringing your attention from the external world towards the inside, enabling you to hear the wisdom of your inner voice.

Dharana Intense concentration allows the rest of your mind to become calm and settled. In dharana, you learn to focus your consciousness on a single point.

Dhyana Very similar to dharana, the seventh limb of yoga encourages you to experience the same awareness you experience with single-pointed concentration, only this time without focusing on anything in particular. In essence...

Samadhi This describes both the process of meditation and the state of bliss that can be achieved from meditation.

Your essential gear
YOGA KIT

You don't need to spend a fortune on yoga kit, but the right props and clothing will make your practice more comfortable and enjoyable

Clothing

Any comfortable clothing that allows you to move your body freely will be fine to practise yoga, although if you want to invest in special gear, there's an abundance of attractive styles and performance fabrics available. Here are a few points to bear in mind to make sure what you wear won't interfere with your home practice.

BRA

Unlike some fitness activities, you don't need extra support to do yoga but if you have a larger bust you may want to wear a close-fitting crop top that covers your whole bust – especially important when you're turning your body upside down! Otherwise, wear your normal bra, or opt for a soft, stretchy bra top.

TOPS

A long, close-fitting top is ideal – loose ones may ride up around your neck when you do inversions, or hide your face in any pose where your head is lower than your hips. If you'd rather not wear figure-hugging t-shirts, layering is another option – wear a thin, lightweight tee over a snug one – or try a baggy t-shirt that has a close fitting band around the hips. Keep an extra layer close by for the beginning and end of the class, when your body will be cooler.

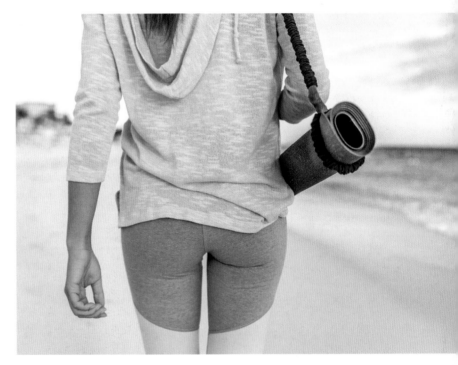

BOTTOMS

Stretchy, close-fitting leggings or capri pants are best as they won't impede your movement and they let you check on the alignment of your legs. Overly loose pants, on the other hand, may get trapped beneath your body as you twist. Avoid thick waistlines, though, or heavy drawstrings at the waist, as they could be uncomfortable when folding forwards or lying on your stomach.

tip

If your hips are tight and you don't have a strap, place a block or cushion underneath each knee.

Props

When you're beginning your yoga journey, props can be really useful for letting you get a feel for a pose before you have full strength or flexibility. Think of them as an extension of your body and a way to experience the benefits of the pose immediately. These are the best props to start with.

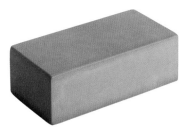

BRICK

Bricks are usually deeper and wider than blocks, often making them more stable and more suitable for weight bearing. Use them for poses such as Pyramid (p83), where you may have more weight travelling through your hands, or to support your knees in poses such as Reclining butterfly (p76).

BORROW: **Find a thick, short book**

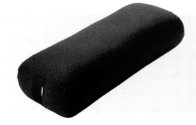

BOLSTER

A bolster is perfect for making your practice more comfortable, and is indispensable for restorative yoga. Bolsters come in cylindrical or rectangular shapes, although you may find the latter more useful as its wider surface makes it ideal to rest your back on.

BORROW: **Grab a couple of firm pillows or long cushions**

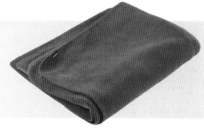

BLANKET

Folded under your shoulders, a firm blanket will protect your neck in Shoulder stand (p118). It will also help open your chest when lying on your back. A blanket is perfect for keeping you warm at the end of your session, in Relaxation pose (p26). Choose a fleece or cotton blanket.

BORROW: **Take one off your bed or use a large throw**

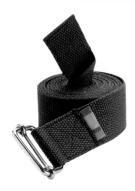

YOGA STRAP

Straps are a great way to experience correct alignment, regardless of your flexibility. Use them as an extension of your arms and wrap one around your feet in Head to knee pose (p52), or use it to help you balance in Boat (p98).

BORROW: **Use a tie or belt**

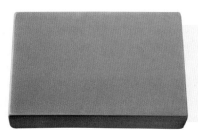

BLOCK

A foam block can be used as an extension of your arms in standing poses such as Standing forward fold (p31), or to support your shoulder in Reclining twist (p34 and p53). One of their most common uses is to sit on it if your spine rounds, such as in Staff pose (p50). Two will be fine to start with (one for each hand).

BORROW: **Find two books of the same thickness**

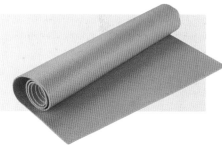

YOGA MAT

A mat helps cushion your joints from hard floors and stops your hands and feet slipping when you're in postures such as Downward dog (p65). Choose the mat's thickness according to your needs. Prices vary from £15 to £100 but you'll get an adequate mat for under £20.

BORROW: **Use a thick cotton rug**

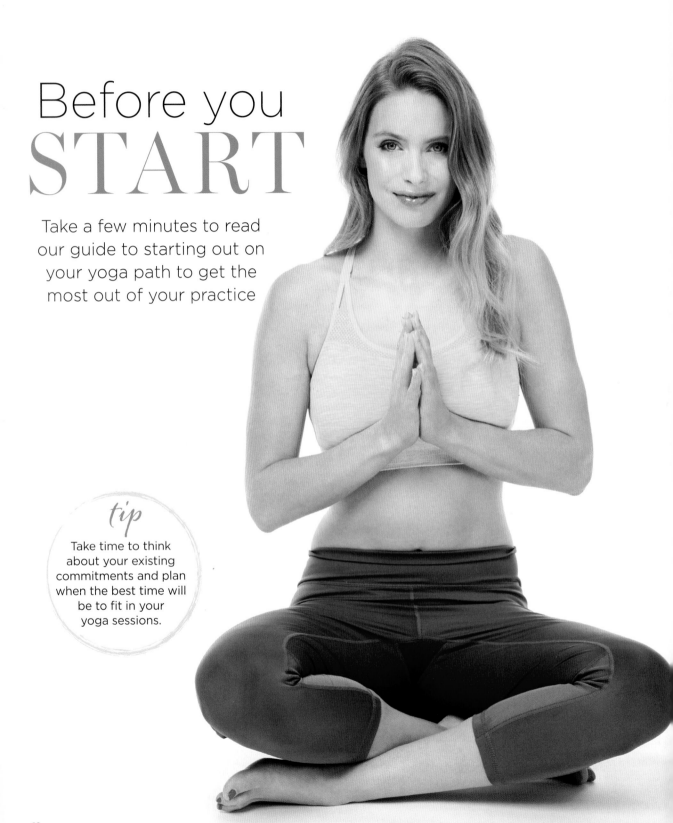

Before you
START

Take a few minutes to read our guide to starting out on your yoga path to get the most out of your practice

tip

Take time to think about your existing commitments and plan when the best time will be to fit in your yoga sessions.

1 Traditionally yoga is practised first thing in the morning, giving you energy, increasing your focus and preparing you for the day ahead. In the evening, a yoga session can help you wind down, let go of the tensions of the day and help you get a good night's sleep. Having a set time that you practise helps you make yoga a regular part of your life, so chose a time that fits in with your other commitments and aim to stick to it as often as you can.

2 It's best to practise yoga on an empty stomach – you'll feel lighter and more agile, and the forward bends and twists, in particular, will be much easier. Aim to practise two to three hours after a meal or, if you prefer to do your yoga session first thing in the morning, have half a banana or an oatcake about 30 minutes beforehand.

3 As with food, don't drink too much water before your yoga session – it will sit heavily on your stomach. Take sips of water during your practice and remember to stay hydrated throughout the day.

4 Create a welcoming environment to practise in. A clear uncluttered space will instantly calm you and put you in the right frame of mind. Make the most of natural light, facing a window if possible, or use soft lighting or scented candles in the evening. You can also use flowers, a statue of a Buddha or a photograph or symbol that has meaning to help you settle into a quiet reflective place inside yourself.

5 Always warm up your body before your main yoga practice, ideally moving your spine in all planes of movement – flexion and extension (forward bends and back bends), a lateral stretch and a twist. The warm-ups in this book each target specific muscles used in that week's sequence, helping to prevent injury, so don't miss out this important stage of your practice.

"Your body is your best teacher, so learn to listen to your body as you practise"

6 Your anatomy will have a big impact on which poses you find easy and which are more challenging. Someone who is hyper-mobile will find it easy to get their heels on the ground in Downward dog pose (p65), for example. Rather than compare yourself with other people, give your attention to the improvements to your own body, and take notice of how your strength and flexibility increases week after week.

7 Remember, your body is your best teacher, so learn to listen to your body as you practise, and trust the messages it gives you, drawing back if a pose feels too strong, lingering a little longer or repeating it if your body is savouring the pose and asking for more.

8 When you begin yoga, little and often is best. If you want to have a daily practice while following this programme, try just doing the warm-ups for the week you are working on. You can include the half and beginner's sun salutes as they are introduced, and can also work on one or two specific poses you'd like to focus on.

9 Focus on your internal experience. Learn to feel a posture from the inside rather than give excessive attention to the way it looks from the outside.

STAY SAFE

● **IF YOU** are pregnant or think you have a health condition that may affect your practice, check with your doctor or a qualified yoga teacher to ensure it is safe for you to practise the postures in this book.

● **ALWAYS LISTEN** to your body. A mild ache while you are in a pose is usually a sign that your body is opening into a stretch, but if you feel a sharp or sudden pain, come out of the asana and try it another day, not going so deeply into the posture.

● **AVOID INVERTED** postures such as Shoulder stand (p118) if you have high blood pressure or are menstruating. Replace them with Reclining wide angle pose (p85).

● **TAKE CARE** of your knees. Keep your knee directly over your ankle in poses such as Crescent (p80), High Lunge (p82) and Extended side angle (p48). Your knee only has about 15 degrees of rotation when in flexion (a bent position). If you find crossed leg positions such as Easy (p24) or Accomplished (p25) poses uncomfortable for your knees, sit on a block or bolster.

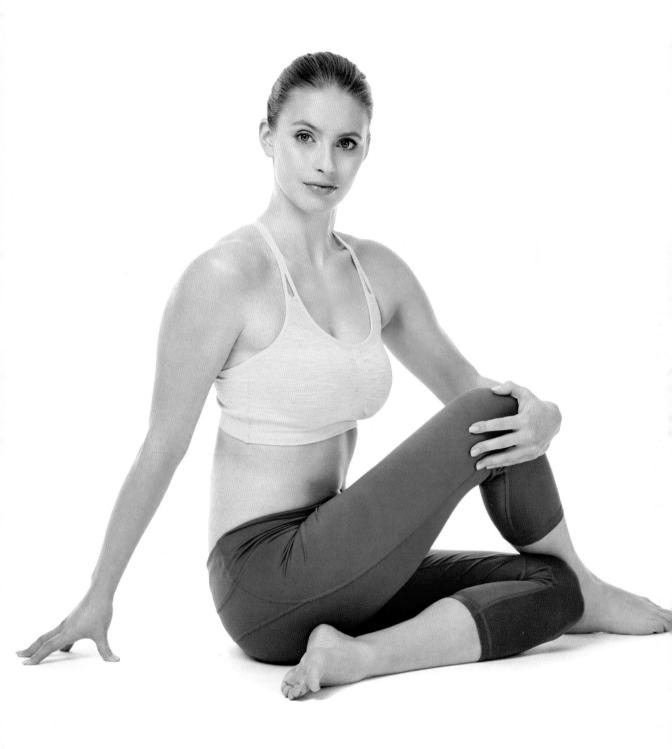

Week 1

Now that you've covered the basics, it's time to get started with your **first yoga lesson**. This week, you'll learn about the importance of the **breath** in yoga and become more aware of your own breathing patterns. We'll also introduce you to **12 foundation poses** that will enable you to practise the techniques you have learnt. Give yourself plenty of time to read through the instructions for each pose **carefully** and try each move before moving on to this week's sequence on page 36.

"WHEN THE BREATH WANDERS

THE MIND IS ALSO UNSTEADY.

BUT WHEN THE BREATH IS CALMED

THE MIND TOO WILL BE STILL AND

THE YOGI ACHIEVES LONG LIFE.

THEREFORE, ONE SHOULD LEARN

TO CONTROL THE BREATH"

Swami Muktibodhananda
(Hatha Yoga Pradipika)

THIS WEEK'S FOCUS

BREATHING WELL

Becoming aware of your breath is central to yoga. Breathing skilfully, and moving with your breath, brings your mind and body into balance and leaves you feeling calm and centred

In your practice this week, unless otherwise instructed, aim to breathe for an equal length on the inhale and exhale, through your nose if you can, as this allows a cleaner, warmer breath, and gives you more control. Let your breath be your guide – if your breathing becomes strained, or you notice you are holding your breath, you're probably working too hard. Ease up a bit and listen to what your body needs. If you are sluggish and not feeling engaged with the postures, breathe in a more conscious way and you'll soon feel more energised and present.

Let your breath instigate movement, inhaling as you unfold your body, lengthen your spine, open your chest or raise your arms. Follow your exhalation when you root into the ground, deepen into a forward fold or release into a twist, each time giving your weight back to the earth that supports you.

If you can, spend some time this week getting to know your breathing habits off the mat. Check-in periodically throughout the day and observe your breath. Try not to change anything – just notice how you are breathing. You may find you're taking shallow rapid breaths from your chest or perhaps you are enjoying slow, deep abdominal breaths. In moments of stress, you may even find you've been holding your breath. Getting to know how you breathe and, over time learning to control it, will benefit your yoga practice immensely – and your life.

Your Week 1 yoga sessions

Each week, we'll give you a suggested plan to follow, but feel free to work in the way that works best for you. You may prefer to do a short 10-minute session every day, or set aside longer chunks of time for a more substantial practice. It's a good idea to practise each pose at least once before completing the class at the end of the chapter, and aim to do the class at least once in the week.

WEEK ONE

NEW POSES

✦ Easy pose
✦ Accomplished pose
✦ Relaxation pose
✦ Cat/Cow
✦ Child's pose
✦ Mountain pose
✦ Extended mountain pose
✦ Standing forward fold
✦ Half standing forward fold
✦ Bridge
✦ Knees to chest
✦ Reclining twist I

NEW SEQUENCE

✦ Half sun salute

SUGGESTED PLAN

Session 1 (20 minutes) Warm-up poses and breathing exercise

Session 2 (20 minutes) Standing poses and Half sun salute

Finish with Relaxation pose

Session 3 (1 hour) Week 1 sequence

EASY POSE
Sukhasana

● Sit on your mat and cross your legs at the shins, so your lower legs are parallel to the front edge of the mat. Use your hands to draw one buttock and then the other away from your mid-line. This will help you root into the ground through your sitting bones.

● Flex your feet to stabilise and protect your knees, then place your hands (or fingertips) either side of your hips, and root down as you draw your navel to your spine and lengthen up out of your pelvis.

● Open your chest, draw your shoulder blades down your back and lift through the crown. Lengthen the back of your neck and softly close your eyes, or gaze a few feet in front of you on the floor.

● Rest your hands on your knees and allow your weight to sink into the floor on each exhale. Let your mind become still.

● Breathe calmly and evenly into your abdomen as long as is comfortable, then gently open your eyes.

GOOD FOR

✦ Grounding and centring
✦ Soothes your nervous system
✦ Calms and settles your mind

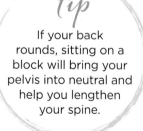

tip
If your back rounds, sitting on a block will bring your pelvis into neutral and help you lengthen your spine.

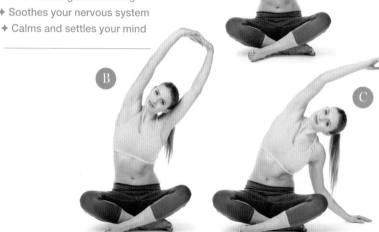

VARIATIONS

Easy pose with side stretch I

From Easy pose, interlace your fingers, turn your palms away from you and straighten your arms, raising them in front of you to chest height. Inhale as you arc your hands overhead (A), then exhale as you reach your arms over to your left (B). Take three deep breaths into your right side body, then inhale to return to centre. Pause, then repeat on the other side.

Easy pose with side stretch II

From Easy pose, rest your left hand on the floor and, on an inhale, raise your right arm out to the side and overhead. Exhale. On your next inhale, reach your arm over to your left (C). Feel the stretch in your right side body without tilting your body forwards. Take three to five breaths then release on an exhale and repeat on the other side.

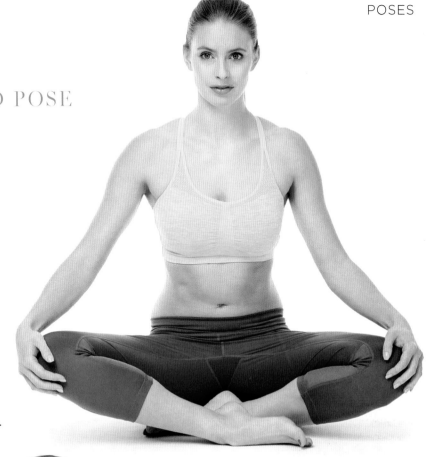

ACCOMPLISHED POSE
Siddhasana

- Sit on your mat with your feet extended in front of you. As with Easy pose (p24), use your hands to draw one buttock and then the other away from your mid-line to help you root into the ground through your sitting bones.
- Take your left heel to your perineum and let your left knee fold out to the side. Bring your right foot in to your left, your right knee releasing outwards, and align your heels. Rest your hands on your knees.
- Feel your sitting bones on the mat, engage your core slightly and open your chest as you draw your shoulder blades down your back and lift through the crown. Rest in the pose for five to 10 breaths then gently release.

tip

If Accomplished pose is more comfortable than Easy pose, swap it whenever Easy pose or variations are used in the **sequences**.

VARIATION
Accomplished pose with twist
Place your left hand on the floor behind your left buttock, fingers pointing backwards, and rest your right palm on the outside of your left knee. Inhale as you root through your sitting bones to lift your spine out of your pelvis.

On an exhale, slowly rotate your spine to the left, moving in a spiral from your waist initially, then your upper body. Inhale, lengthen through the crown of your head, exhale further into the twist. If comfortable for your neck, turn your head to look over your left shoulder.

Inhale back to the centre and repeat on the other side.

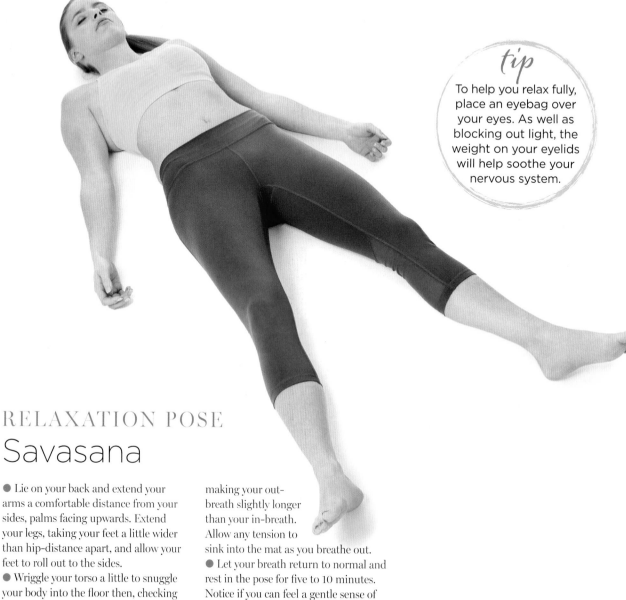

RELAXATION POSE
Savasana

● Lie on your back and extend your arms a comfortable distance from your sides, palms facing upwards. Extend your legs, taking your feet a little wider than hip-distance apart, and allow your feet to roll out to the sides.

● Wriggle your torso a little to snuggle your body into the floor then, checking that your arms and legs are symmetrical, rest your head on the centre of the back of your skull. Gently close your eyes.

● Begin to allow any tension in your body to seep away into the floor, consciously letting go on each exhalation.

● Breathe softly and evenly into your belly, letting your eyelids be heavy, your jaw soft and your belly relaxed. Rest for a few moments, then let your breath become a little slower and deeper,

making your out-breath slightly longer than your in-breath. Allow any tension to sink into the mat as you breathe out.

● Let your breath return to normal and rest in the pose for five to 10 minutes. Notice if you can feel a gentle sense of expansion as you inhale, and a feeling of softening as you exhale.

● To come out of the pose, slowly wriggle your fingers and toes. Slide your arms out to the sides and overhead, and gently stretch your body from your feet to your fingertips. Slowly bring your knees to your chest, roll over to your right hand side and rest for few moments. Then use your left hand to help you come up to sitting.

GOOD FOR

✦ Calming your mind
✦ Balancing your mind, body and spirit
✦ Rejuvenating
✦ Reducing fatigue

CAT/COW POSE
Marjaryasana/Bitilasana

Cat

● Come onto all fours, with your shoulders directly above your wrists and your hips directly above your knees. Spread your fingers wide, middle fingers pointing forwards. Keep your shins and feet parallel and rest the tops of your toes on the floor. Bring your neck in line with your spine and direct your gaze towards the floor.

● Inhale, then, as you exhale, press into the ground with your hands and the tops of your toes as you release your head and tailbone to the floor and lift your spine towards the ceiling.
This is Cat pose.

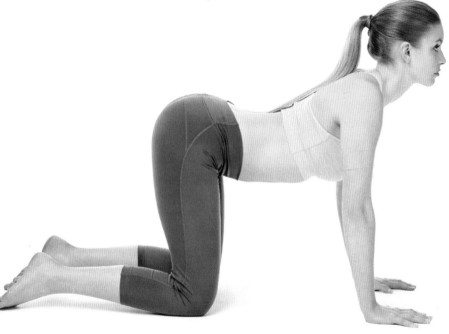

Cow

● On your next inhale, tilt your tailbone up and release your spine down into a gentle backbend. Draw your shoulders down your back, take your chest forwards and up and gently raise your head, gazing softly forwards. This is Cow pose.

● Continue alternating between Cat and Cow poses, instigating the movement from your pelvis and following the natural pattern of your breath. Move vertebra by vertebra in a slow and fluid way for one to two minutes.

GOOD FOR

✦ Opening your chest

✦ Mobilising your spine

✦ Gently massaging your abdominal organs

✦ Teaching you to move with the breath

27

EXTENDED CHILD'S POSE
Utthita balasana

● Kneel on your mat, then using your hands to help you balance, take your knees wide apart and bring your big toes together, letting your heels fall out to the sides as you sit back on the soles of your feet. Rest your palms on your thighs. Take a couple of breaths.

● Inhale as you root into your sitting bones to lengthen your spine. On an exhale, slowly walk your hands forwards, as you lower your torso between your thighs.

● Take your hands shoulder-width apart, palms down, fingers spread. Root your hands into the floor, keeping your elbows off the mat, then slide your shoulder blades down your back and your tailbone towards your heels.

● Exhale and lower your head, gently resting your forehead on the floor, a block or a bolster. Softly close your eyes.

● Breathe deeply and evenly into your back body for five to 10 breaths, sinking deeper into the mat each time your exhale.

● On an exhale, use your hands to gently bring you up to a comfortable seated position.

GOOD FOR
✦ Relieving stress and fatigue
✦ Encouraging introspection
✦ Nurturing
✦ Calming

tip

If your spine rounds too much, come back up to kneeling, put your thumbs in your hip creases and push down and back to help you fold from the hips.

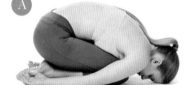

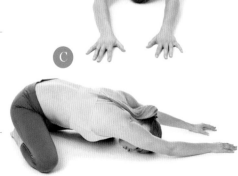

VARIATIONS
Child's pose
From Extended child's pose, take your hands beside your hips, palms facing upwards. Rest your forehead on the floor or on a block, or turn your head to rest on one side (A), remembering to create space around your neck by drawing your shoulders away from your ears. Rest here for up to five minutes, turning your head half-way through if you've chosen to rest on one side.

Extended child's pose with side stretch
From Extended child's pose, inhale, ground your hands on the mat, raise your head and walk your hands round to your right. On an exhale, release your left hip back onto your left foot (B). Breathe into your left side body and feel the expansion of your ribs. Take two more breaths here, then exhale to walk your hands back to the centre and repeat on the other side (C).

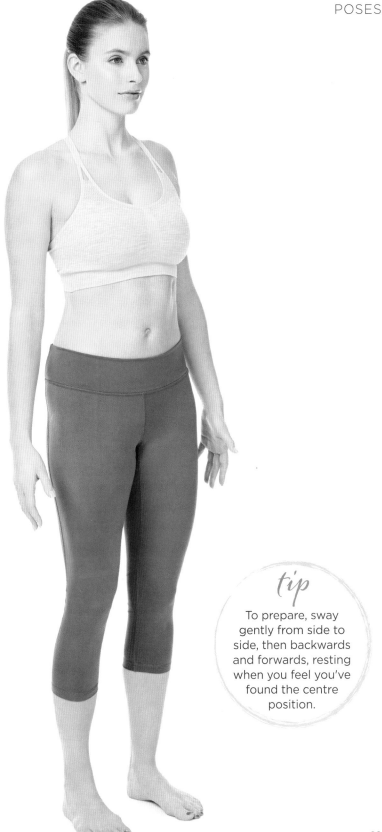

MOUNTAIN POSE
Tadasana

● Place your feet shoulder-width apart, inner edges parallel. Balance your weight evenly over each foot, spread your toes and root through the base of your big and little toes. Lift your inner arches by drawing your ankles away from each other.

● Align your knees over your ankles and your pelvis over your knees. Relax your buttocks and allow your tail and sitting bones to release to the floor. Breathe deeply and evenly.

● Draw your navel towards your spine and release your shoulders down your back. Let your arms hang loosely at your sides, then gently extend through to your fingertips. Release and lengthen the back of your neck.

● As you inhale, ground through your feet and feel the corresponding lift in your spine as you lengthen through to the crown of your head, maintaining the length in your torso when you exhale. Let your breath be gentle, feeling the length and lightness of each in-breath, a sense of grounding and stability on the out-breath. Rest in the pose for up to one minute.

GOOD FOR

✦ Grounding

✦ Steadying the breath

tip

To prepare, sway gently from side to side, then backwards and forwards, resting when you feel you've found the centre position.

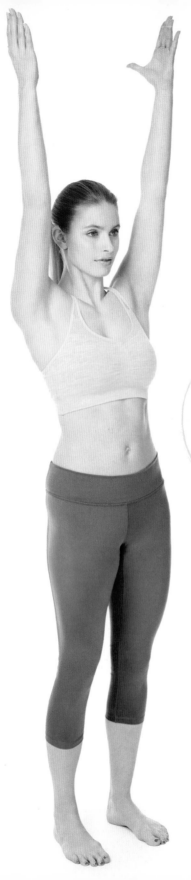

EXTENDED MOUNTAIN POSE
Urdhva hastasana

● From Mountain pose (p29), inhale and root though your feet as you lift your waist out of your hips to lengthen your spine. At the same time, turn your palms outwards and extend your arms in a large circle out to the sides of your body and overhead. Your palms are now parallel and facing each other.

● As you exhale, draw your shoulders down your spine. This will create space around your neck. Gently drop your chin.

● Continue to ground through your feet. Draw your leg muscles in to your bones, your navel towards your spine and your lower ribs in slightly.

● On each inhale, root down to lift through your crown and extend right to the ends of your fingertips at the same time as drawing your arms into your arm sockets. On each exhale, visualise your breath travelling down your body and through your feet.

● Keep your gaze soft and take five to 10 deep breaths, releasing your arms as you exhale.

GOOD FOR
✦ Grounding
✦ Energising
✦ Stretching your side body
✦ Aiding deeper breathing

tip

To develop extension in your arms, interlace your fingers, palms facing the ceiling, and reach up as you draw your shoulders down your back.

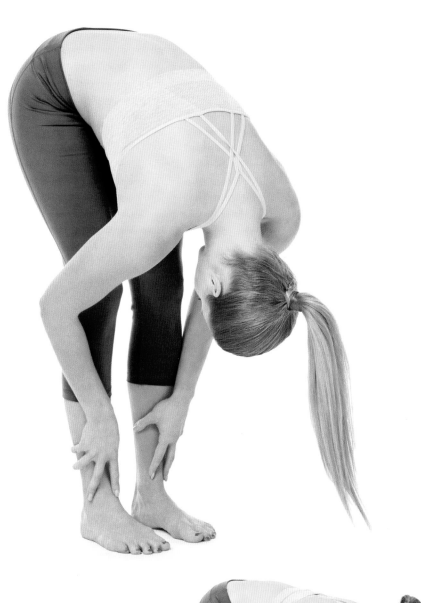

STANDING FORWARD FOLD
Uttanasana

● Stand with your feet hip-width apart and place your hands to your hips. On an inhale, ground through your feet and see if you can lengthen your spine out of your pelvis. On an exhale, slowly fold forwards from your hips, with a flat back. When your spine is parallel to the floor, let your pelvis come into neutral.

● With a slight bend in your knees, inhale and lengthen your spine once more, then, as you exhale, continue folding and allow your chest to rest on your thighs. Bend your knees as much as you need. Release your arms and rest your hands on your shins, ankles or the floor.

● Keeping your knees bent, let your upper body relax fully, then take your tailbone towards the ceiling and allow your head to release closer to the floor.

● On each in-breath, feel your spine lengthening; on each out-breath, fold a little deeper. Surrender to gravity, breathing softly and evenly for several breaths, then inhale to gently uncurl your spine to return to standing.

GOOD FOR
✦ Calming the sympathetic nervous system
✦ Relieving fatigue
✦ Reducing insomnia

VARIATION
Half standing forward fold
From Standing forward fold, knees bent or straight, place your hands a few inches in front of your feet. Inhale as you lengthen your crown away from your tailbone to come up to a flat back. Root through your hands and feet and draw your shoulder blades down your spine. Take five deep breaths and release back into standing forward fold.

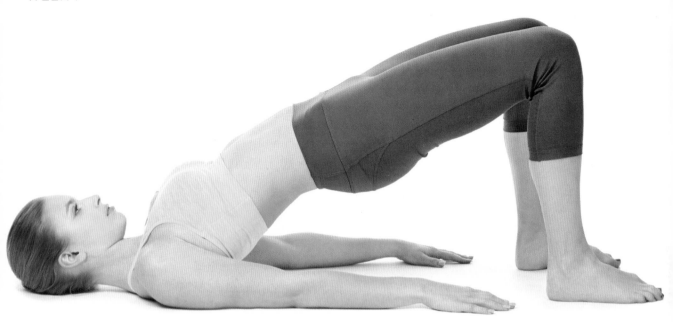

BRIDGE
Setu bandha sarvangasana

● Lie on your back with your knees bent, feet on the floor, directly beneath your knees hip-distance apart and parallel. Rest your arms by your sides, palms facing down.

● On an inhale, spread your toes, ground through your feet and, as you exhale, tilt your tailbone upwards to gently peel your spine away from the floor, one vertebra at a time.

● Keeping your thighs parallel, with your knees hip-distance apart, continue to root your feet into the ground. This will help you lift your chest upwards. Roll your shoulders up, back and down, then lengthen the back of your neck.

● Take five deep breaths into your abdomen then, on an exhale, slowly uncurl your spine, one vertebra at a time, to rest on the floor. Pause for a moment, then when you feel ready, repeat once or twice more.

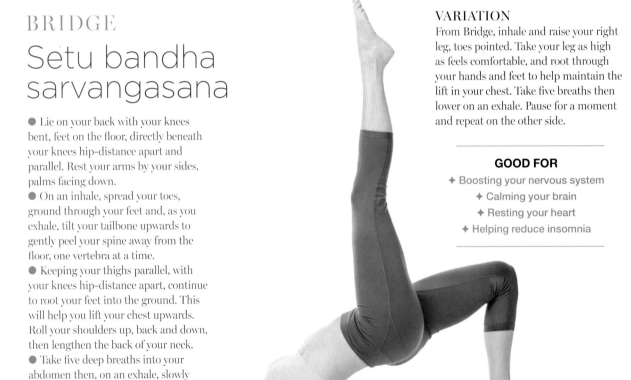

VARIATION
From Bridge, inhale and raise your right leg, toes pointed. Take your leg as high as feels comfortable, and root through your hands and feet to help maintain the lift in your chest. Take five breaths then lower on an exhale. Pause for a moment and repeat on the other side.

GOOD FOR
✦ Boosting your nervous system
✦ Calming your brain
✦ Resting your heart
✦ Helping reduce insomnia

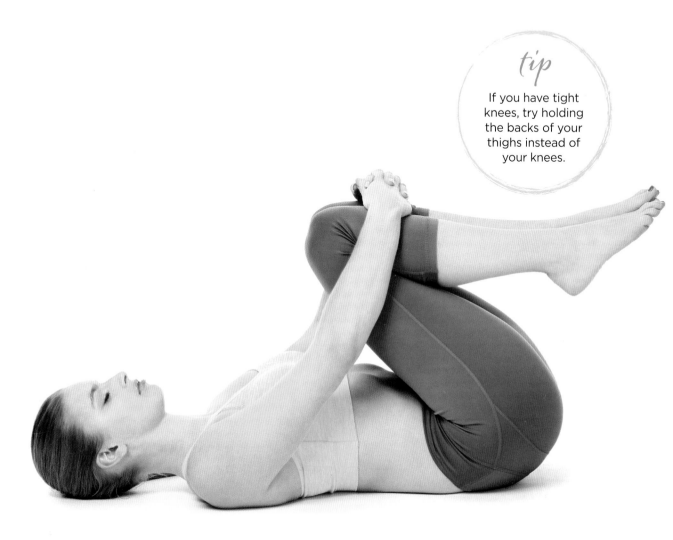

tip

If you have tight knees, try holding the backs of your thighs instead of your knees.

KNEES TO CHEST POSE

Apasana

● Lie on your back and take a few moments to become centred.

● Gently close your eyes then, on an exhale, bring your legs together and draw your knees in to your chest. Wrap your arms around your shins, just below your knees and, if comfortable, hug them in to your chest.

● On each inhale, see if you can notice your back expanding, on each exhale gently softening. Allow your knees to drift forwards slightly as you breathe in, hug them in closer as you breathe out.

● Take 10 to 20 deep breaths, sensing the gentle expansion and contraction of your body. Then, if comfortable, softly sway from side to side to give your lower back a gentle massage.

GOOD FOR

✦ Stretching your spine
✦ Deeply relaxing
✦ Aiding sleep

RECLINING TWIST I
Supta parivartanasana I

● Lie on your back, gently close your eyes and take a few moments to centre yourself, allowing your breath to deepen and your heartbeat to become slower. When you feel ready, move into the pose.
● To begin, lift your buttocks and shift them slightly to the right. This will help you maintain a healthy alignment of your spine.
● Hug both your knees to your chest, using your forearms to bring them in close. Draw your shoulder blades down your back, and take a few breaths into your belly.

● When you feel ready, release your hands and inhale. As you exhale, gently allow your legs to release over to your left, aiming to keep your right shoulder as close to the floor as possible. Extend your arms out to the sides, shoulder height and palms facing upwards. If comfortable, turn your head to look to the left.
● Breathe deeply into your right side, enjoying the stretch for five to 10 deep breaths, then slowly inhale back to centre and repeat on the other side.

tip

If your knees don't manage to reach the floor, rest them on a block or bolster instead for the same effect.

GOOD FOR

✦ Reducing stress
✦ Releasing tension in your spine
✦ Opening your chest
✦ Easing stiffness in your lower back

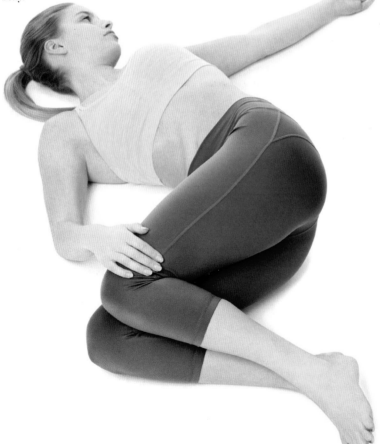

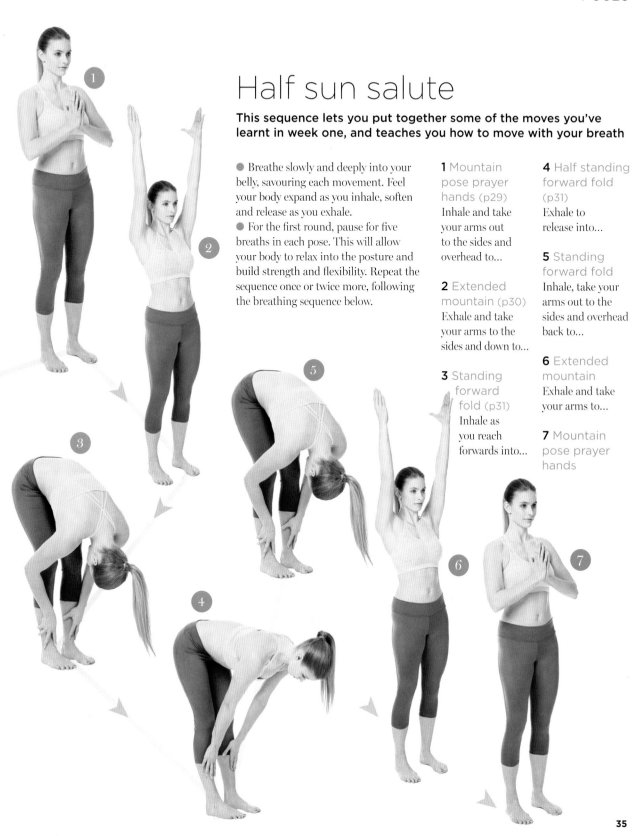

Half sun salute

This sequence lets you put together some of the moves you've learnt in week one, and teaches you how to move with your breath

● Breathe slowly and deeply into your belly, savouring each movement. Feel your body expand as you inhale, soften and release as you exhale.

● For the first round, pause for five breaths in each pose. This will allow your body to relax into the posture and build strength and flexibility. Repeat the sequence once or twice more, following the breathing sequence below.

1 Mountain pose prayer hands (p29) Inhale and take your arms out to the sides and overhead to...

2 Extended mountain (p30) Exhale and take your arms to the sides and down to...

3 Standing forward fold (p31) Inhale as you reach forwards into...

4 Half standing forward fold (p31) Exhale to release into...

5 Standing forward fold Inhale, take your arms out to the sides and overhead back to...

6 Extended mountain Exhale and take your arms to...

7 Mountain pose prayer hands

THE SEQUENCE

This week we focus on learning to breathe well. When you breathe properly, you breathe life into your yoga postures

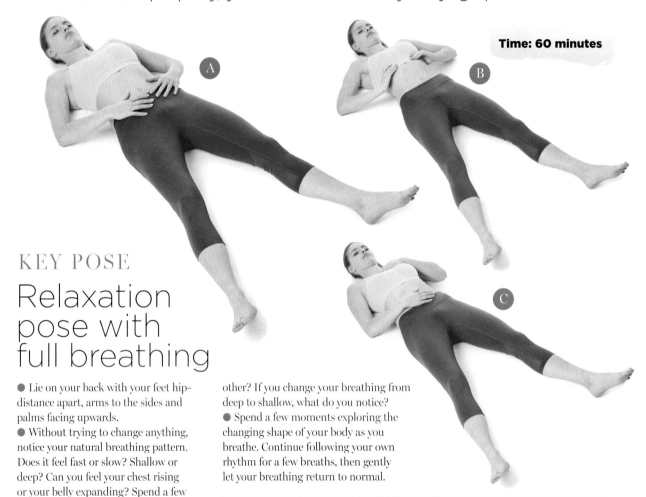

Time: 60 minutes

KEY POSE

Relaxation pose with full breathing

● Lie on your back with your feet hip-distance apart, arms to the sides and palms facing upwards.

● Without trying to change anything, notice your natural breathing pattern. Does it feel fast or slow? Shallow or deep? Can you feel your chest rising or your belly expanding? Spend a few moments just observing your breath.

● Next, rest your hands below your abdomen, fingertips touching (A). Do you feel your belly rising as you inhale, falling as you exhale? Slide your hands to your side ribs (B). Can you sense any movement beneath your hands? Finally, place one hand on your chest with the other on your abdomen (C). Is one hand moving more than the other? If you change your breathing from deep to shallow, what do you notice?

● Spend a few moments exploring the changing shape of your body as you breathe. Continue following your own rhythm for a few breaths, then gently let your breathing return to normal.

> *tip*
>
> In his book *Yoga Sutras*, the ancient sage Patanjali defined yoga as 'Yogas citta vrtti nirodhah' or 'Yoga is calming the fluctuations of the mind'.
> As you begin your first yoga class in this programme, if you notice thoughts coming into your mind, such as 'Am I doing it right?' or 'I must remember the next pose', simply take your attention back to your breath. Let your thoughts gently recede along with each exhalation.

ARRIVE/PREPARE

RELAXATION POSE (p26)

Follow the instructions for full yogic breath

TAKE FIVE BREATHS IN EACH POSE UNLESS OTHERWISE STATED

SIDE RIBS
Focus on expanding your side ribs

EASY POSE (p24)

Breathe into your belly for one to two minutes to quieten your mind

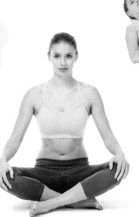

CHEST
Make your out-breath longer than your in-breath

BELLY
Observe the rise and fall of your abdomen

WARM-UP

1
EASY POSE, ARMS OVERHEAD (p24)

CHEST
Inhale to take your hands overhead, exhale to reach to the side

2
CAT/COW (p27)
10 breaths

BACK
Exhale as you arc your spine

CHEST
Inhale as you lift your chest

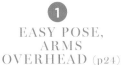
Move with your breath

4
ACCOMPLISHED POSE WITH TWIST (p25)

ABDOMEN
Inhale to lengthen, exhale to twist

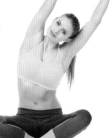

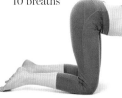

3
CHILD'S POSE (p28)

BACK
Breathe into your back body

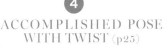

STANDING

1

STANDING FORWARD FOLD (p31)

KNEES
Keep a bend in your knees if needed

2

HALF STANDING FORWARD FOLD (p31)

BACK
Lengthen from your tailbone to your crown

3

MOUNTAIN POSE (p29)

FEET
Sway from side to side until you find the central position

4

EXTENDED MOUNTAIN POSE (p30)

SHOULDERS
Keep your shoulders down as you lift through to your fingertips

5

HALF SUN SALUTE (x3)(p35)

CHEST
Remember to move from your breath

PAGE 35

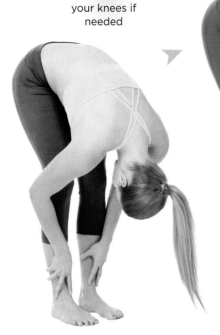

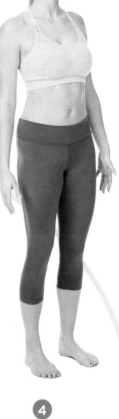

SITTING

1

EXTENDED CHILD'S POSE (p28)

KNEES
Take your knees wide

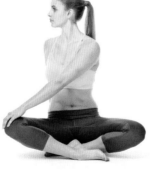

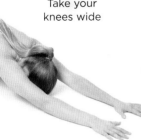

3

BRIDGE (p32)

CHEST
Inhale to lift, exhale to lower

2

ACCOMPLISHED POSE, WITH TWIST (p25)

NECK
If comfortable, turn your head to look over your shoulder

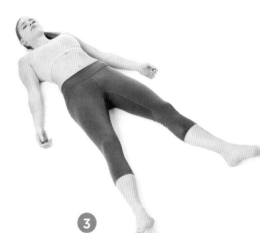

COOL DOWN/RELAXATION

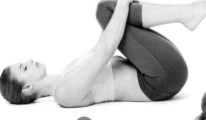

Note ....
Easy pose and Accomplished pose are interchangeable. Use whichever one suits your body most.

1

KNEES TO CHEST (p33)

TORSO
Gently rock from side to side

tip
Your body will cool down rapidly once you are in Relaxation pose. Have a blanket or extra layer close by to cover yourself with.

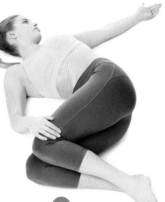

2

LYING TWIST (p34)

SHOULDERS
Aim to keep both shoulders on the floor

3

RELAXATION POSE (p26)

Rest for five minutes

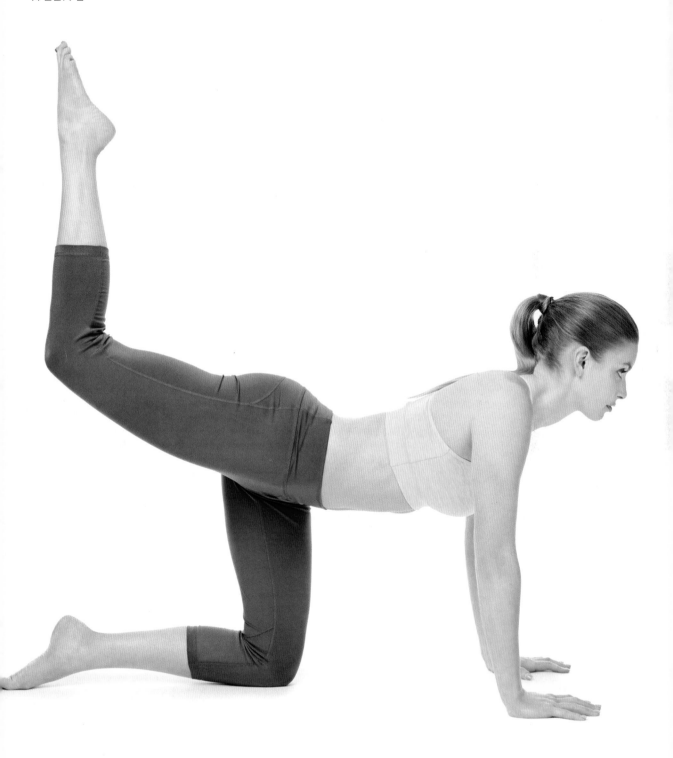

Week 2

Congratulations on completing your first week of yoga! Now it's time to build on your understanding of moving with the breath by learning how to create a strong base in your yoga postures. Whatever part of your body is touching the floor will **form your foundation** and make the pose both stable and dynamic. Over the following pages we'll show you how to use your feet, hands and sitting bones to **maximise the benefits** you experience in each pose, then put it together in a sequence on p68.

"THE MIRACLE IS NOT TO WALK ON WATER. THE MIRACLE IS TO WALK ON THE GREEN EARTH, DWELLING DEEPLY IN THE PRESENT MOMENT AND FEELING TRULY ALIVE"

Thich Nhat Hanh
Zen master and spiritual leader

THIS WEEK'S FOCUS

BEING GROUNDED

Just as the strength of a building is determined by its foundations, the quality of your contact with the ground will be reflected in your yoga postures. Use the following techniques to create strong yoga foundations

Feet: throughout this book we'll be referring to pada bandha or foot lock. To engage pada bandha, stand with the inner edges of your feet parallel and roughly hip-distance apart. Spread your toes wide, and root the base of your big and little toes into the ground (try lifting your three centre toes to help you get a sense of your big and little toes pressing downwards, then release them back down onto the floor). If you imagine your feet as rectangles, make sure your weight is evenly distributed into the four corners of each foot, then raise your inner arches, by drawing your ankles away from the mid-line. You'll use pada bandha in all standing poses, so spend a bit of time this week getting to know how it feels.

Hands: hasta bandha is a similar technique to pada bandha, this time applied to your hands. To practise hand lock, come onto all fours and place your hands on the floor in front of you, shoulder-width apart and middle finger pointing forwards. Spread your fingers and root through the base of your thumb and index finger. Press through all your fingers and thumbs, to slightly raise the centre of your palm – a bit like a suction effect. Don't worry if it doesn't come easily at first, focus on rooting through your fingers initially and the rest will come over time. You'll see a big difference in poses such as Cat/Cow (p27) and Downward dog (p65) when you use hasta bandha.

Your Week 2 yoga sessions

As before, you can fit the poses and sequence around your other commitments, or follow the recommendations below. Try and do each pose at least once before you tackle this week's class, so you don't have to interrupt the flow by having to look closely at the form guides. Set aside time for this week's key pose – an in-depth look at Mountain pose. Whether working on your own or following the plan, always finish with Relaxation pose (p26).

WEEK TWO

NEW POSES

✦ Tiger
✦ Side gate
✦ Warrior II
✦ Triangle
✦ Extended side angle
✦ Wide leg standing forward fold
✦ Staff pose
✦ Sage pose
✦ Head to knee pose
✦ Lying twist II

SUGGESTED PLAN

Session 1 (25 minutes) Tiger, Side gate, key pose, Warrior II, Triangle and Extended side angle

Session 2 (15 minutes) Wide leg standing forward fold, seated poses and Lying twist II

Session 3 (1 hour) Week 2 sequence

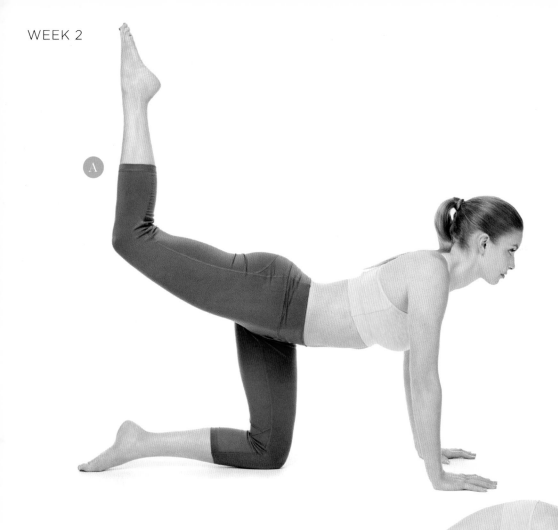

TIGER
Vyaghrasana

● Come onto all fours, with your wrists directly beneath your shoulders, your knees directly beneath your hips, tops of your feet on the floor. Spread your fingers, middle fingers pointing forwards.

● On an inhale, lift your head and chest as you stretch your right leg back and up, bending your knee and pointing your toes towards the ceiling. Keep length in your neck by drawing your shoulders down your spine. Gaze softly forwards (A). Pause for a moment then, as you exhale, bring your knee down and forwards, tucking it under your body and towards your nose as you simultaneously lower your head and arc your spine in an upwards movement. Pause (B).

● Continue alternating between these two poses, timing them with your breath, for 10 to 20 breaths, then repeat on the other leg.

GOOD FOR
✦ Boosting spinal flexibility
✦ Opening your hips
✦ Stimulating circulation
✦ Toning your spinal nerves

WARM-UP

SIDE GATE POSE

Parighasana

● Come onto all fours, with your wrists directly beneath your shoulders, your knees directly beneath your hips, tops of your feet on the floor. Spread your fingers, middle fingers pointing forwards and root through the base of your thumb and index finger.

● Extend your right leg behind you and place your foot flat on the ground, parallel with the short end of your mat and directly behind your left foot. Your right hip will naturally rotate upwards. Pivot on your left knee to take your left foot behind you,

so that your lower leg is parallel to the short end of your mat.

● Rooting through your left hand, inhale as you take your right hand forwards and overhead, alongside your right ear, keeping space around your neck.

● Ground through the outside edge of your right foot, extend your torso out of your hips and feel the stretch all the way from your right toes to your right fingertips.

● Breathe into your side body for five breaths, then gently release on an exhale and repeat on the other side.

GOOD FOR

✦ Toning your abdominal muscles
✦ Boosting spinal flexibility
✦ Aiding breathing capacity
✦ Aiding digestion

tip

If the Side gate pose is too uncomfortable for your knee, fold your mat double, lengthwise.

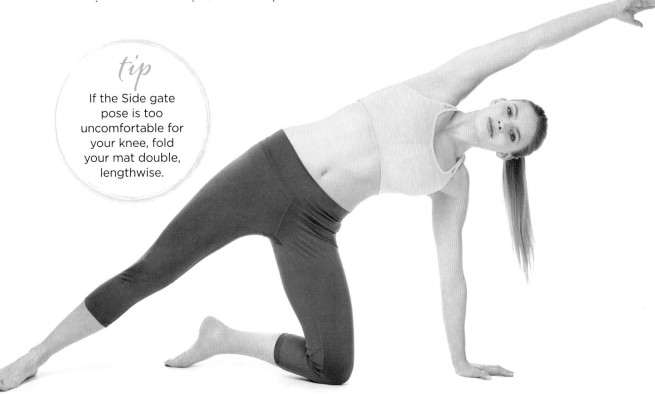

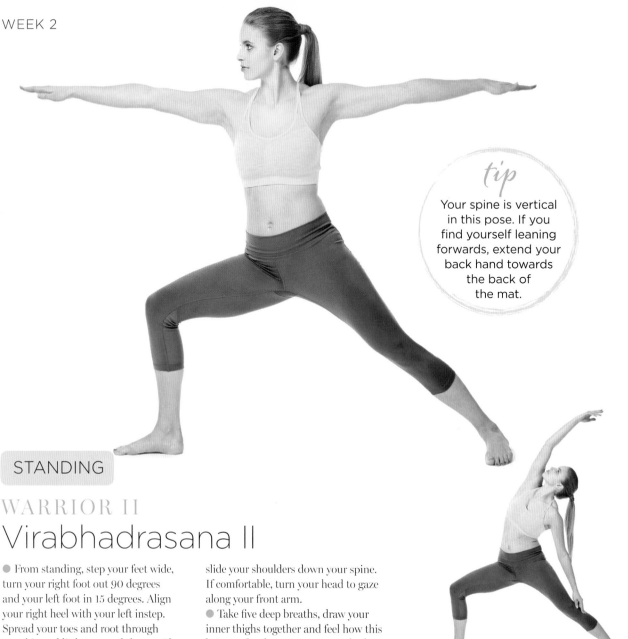

tip
Your spine is vertical in this pose. If you find yourself leaning forwards, extend your back hand towards the back of the mat.

STANDING

WARRIOR II
Virabhadrasana II

● From standing, step your feet wide, turn your right foot out 90 degrees and your left foot in 15 degrees. Align your right heel with your left instep. Spread your toes and root through your big and little toes and the outside edge of your left foot.

● Balance your weight evenly between both feet and check that your pelvis is in neutral and facing the long side of your mat. Inhale and raise your arms to the sides, palms down, and lengthen right through to your fingertips.

● On an exhale, bend your right leg to take your knee directly above your ankle, keeping a micro-bend in your left leg.

● Breathing evenly, draw your navel to your spine, open your chest and slide your shoulders down your spine. If comfortable, turn your head to gaze along your front arm.

● Take five deep breaths, draw your inner thighs together and feel how this brings a freedom to your upper body.

● Gently lower your arms on an exhale and step your feet together. Pause for a moment then repeat on the other side.

GOOD FOR
✦ Focus and determination
✦ Strengthening your legs
✦ Grounding
✦ Helping you connect to your strength

VARIATION
Reverse warrior
From Warrior II, inhale as you slide your back arm down your back thigh, and raise your front arm overhead, gently arching your spine laterally. Root your feet down and lift your torso up on each inhale, feeling your side body open and, as you exhale, arc a little further into the backbend. Take five breaths, then change sides.

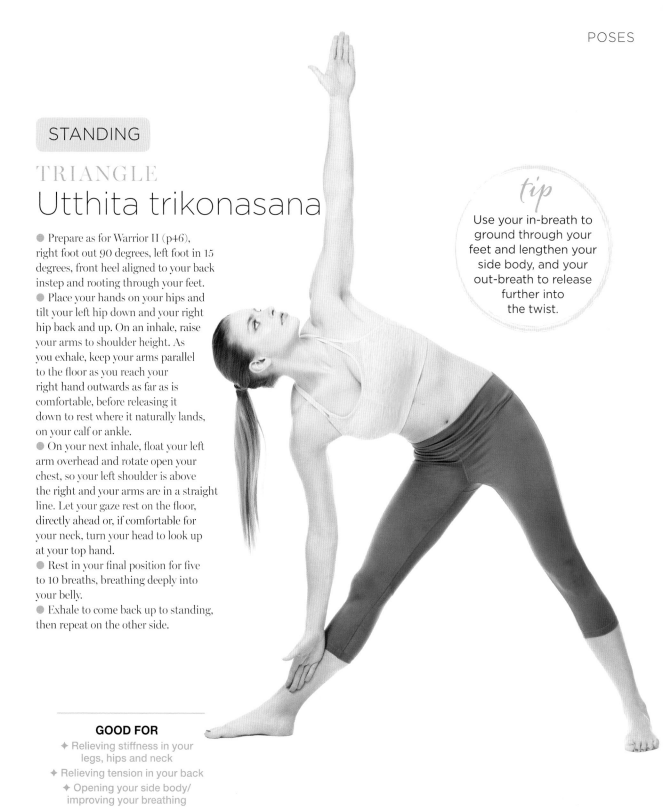

STANDING

TRIANGLE
Utthita trikonasana

● Prepare as for Warrior II (p46), right foot out 90 degrees, left foot in 15 degrees, front heel aligned to your back instep and rooting through your feet.

● Place your hands on your hips and tilt your left hip down and your right hip back and up. On an inhale, raise your arms to shoulder height. As you exhale, keep your arms parallel to the floor as you reach your right hand outwards as far as is comfortable, before releasing it down to rest where it naturally lands, on your calf or ankle.

● On your next inhale, float your left arm overhead and rotate open your chest, so your left shoulder is above the right and your arms are in a straight line. Let your gaze rest on the floor, directly ahead or, if comfortable for your neck, turn your head to look up at your top hand.

● Rest in your final position for five to 10 breaths, breathing deeply into your belly.

● Exhale to come back up to standing, then repeat on the other side.

tip

Use your in-breath to ground through your feet and lengthen your side body, and your out-breath to release further into the twist.

GOOD FOR
✦ Relieving stiffness in your legs, hips and neck
✦ Relieving tension in your back
✦ Opening your side body/ improving your breathing
✦ Easing menstrual symptoms

EXTENDED SIDE ANGLE POSE
Uttitha parsvakonasana

● Step your feet wide and turn your right foot out 90°, your left foot in 15°. Align your right heel to your left instep and root through your toes and outer edge of the left foot.

● Balance your weight evenly between both feet, inhale and raise your arms to the sides, shoulder-height.

● Exhale, bend your right knee over your ankle, keeping a micro-bend in your left leg as you take your right forearm to your thigh and your left hand to your left hip. Tilt your tailbone towards your back heel and rotate your chest upwards and open.

● Then, on an inhale, sweep your left arm overhead and alongside your ear, palm facing down.

● Ground through the outer edge of your back foot to lengthen your entire left side body, from your foot through to your left fingertips. Gaze at the floor or, if comfortable for your neck, your upper hand.

● Take five deep breaths into your belly, savouring the stretch. When you feel ready, exhale and return to standing. Pause, then repeat on the other side.

GOOD FOR
✦ Grounding
✦ Strengthening your legs
✦ Supporting deeper breathing
✦ Aiding balance

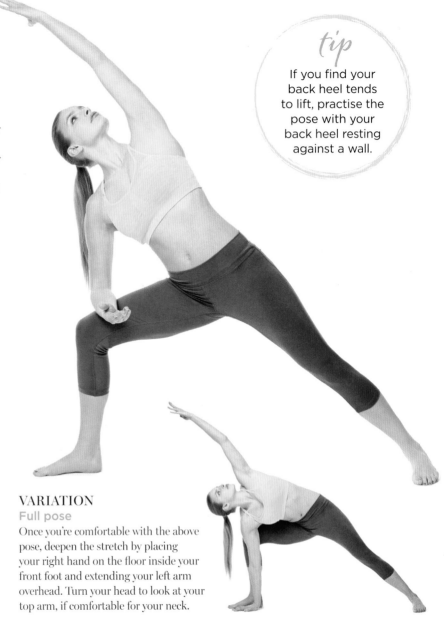

tip
If you find your back heel tends to lift, practise the pose with your back heel resting against a wall.

VARIATION
Full pose
Once you're comfortable with the above pose, deepen the stretch by placing your right hand on the floor inside your front foot and extending your left arm overhead. Turn your head to look at your top arm, if comfortable for your neck.

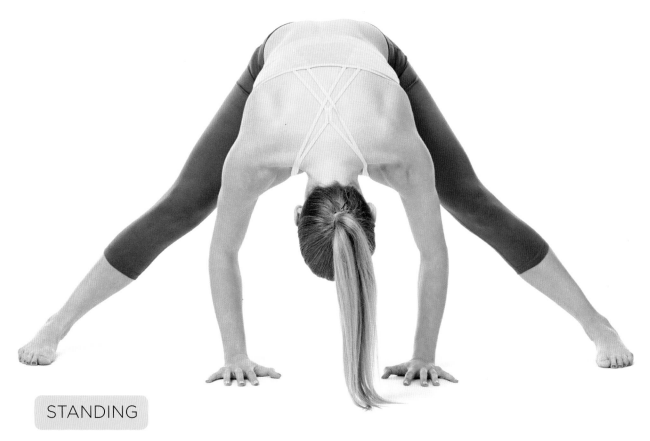

STANDING

WIDE LEGGED STANDING FORWARD FOLD

WIDE LEGGED STANDING FORWARD FOLD
Prasarita padottanasana

● Step your feet wide, inner edges parallel, toes spread and turned slightly inwards, arches lifted. Anchor the outer edges of your feet into the mat.

● Rest your hands on your hips and, on an inhale, root through your feet to lengthen your spine. As you exhale, fold forwards from your hips with a flat back, to take your spine horizontal to the floor.

● Place your hands on the floor beneath your shoulders, then continue lengthening your spine as you inhale, folding deeper as you exhale, allowing the crown of your head to slowly edge closer to the mat.

● Draw up your kneecaps and engage your thighs, turning your inner thighs in slightly to open your sitting bones. Move your hands between your feet, fingers spread wide and forearms vertical, and let your neck and head release towards the floor. Root your hands into the mat to lift your shoulders and create space around your neck.

● Breathe deeply and evenly for five to 10 breaths then, taking your hands back to your hips, inhale to come back up to standing.

GOOD FOR
✦ Resting your heart
✦ Calming and cooling your mind
✦ Removing fatigue
✦ Increasing blood flow to your head

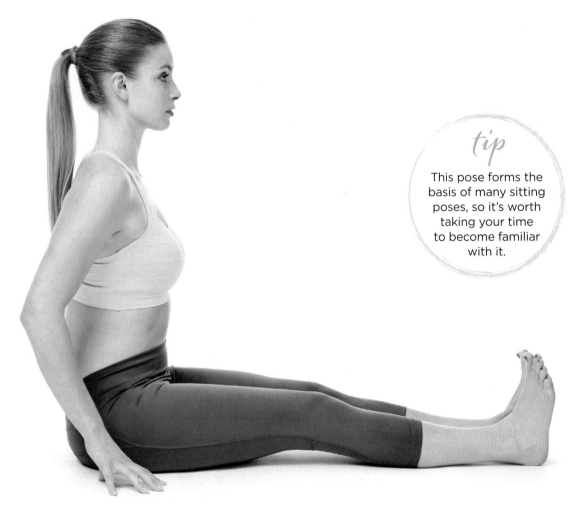

tip

This pose forms the basis of many sitting poses, so it's worth taking your time to become familiar with it.

STAFF POSE

Dandasana

● Sit with your legs straight out in front of you, feet together, ankles flexed and toes pointing to the ceiling. Rest your hands or fingertips on the floor beside your hips, fingers spread and fingertips facing forwards.

● Check that your knees are facing directly upwards and your feet are balanced on the centre of your heels, then when you feel ready, extend through the balls of your feet, spread your toes and reach through the base of your big and little toes. Lift your arches and draw the outside edges of your feet slightly towards your body.

● Roll your inner thighs downwards and inwards, to open your sacrum, and gently shift your weight slightly forwards, to rest on the front of your sitting bones.

● With your pelvis in neutral, root through your hands to extend out of your pelvis, draw your navel to your spine and draw your shoulder blades down your back. Lengthen the back of your neck and extend through the crown of your head.

● Breathe into your belly for five to 10 breaths then gently release.

GOOD FOR

✦ Focusing your mind
✦ Alleviating fatigue
✦ Strengthening your back
✦ Strengthening your core

SITTING

SAGE POSE (STAGE ONE)
Marichyasana

● From Staff pose (p50), bend your left knee and place your foot a hand's distance from your right thigh.
● Inhale and lift your left arm overhead, then as you exhale, twist your body towards the right and wrap your left arm around your left knee. Place your right hand behind you resting on your fingertips or the palm of your hand.

● Take 10 breaths, lengthening your spine on each inhalation, twisting a little deeper on each exhalation. Keep your chest open and your shoulders drawing down your back. If comfortable, turn your head to gaze over your right shoulder.
● When you are ready, inhale, then exhale to return to centre and repeat on the other side.

tip
Keep the muscles of your straight leg engaged, making sure your toes point directly up to the ceiling.

GOOD FOR
✦ Toning your abdominals
✦ Stimulating your digestion
✦ Strengthening your spine

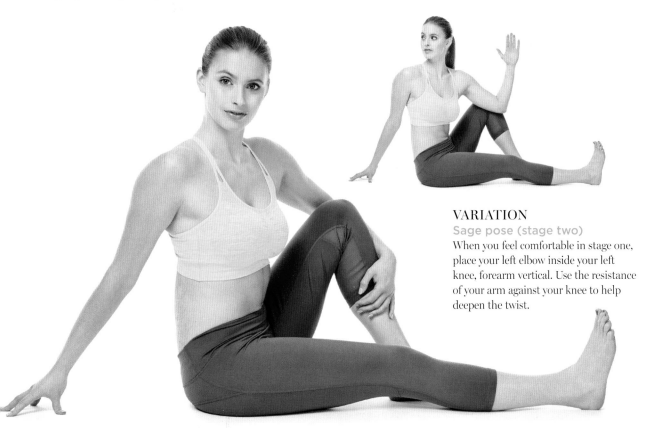

VARIATION
Sage pose (stage two)
When you feel comfortable in stage one, place your left elbow inside your left knee, forearm vertical. Use the resistance of your arm against your knee to help deepen the twist.

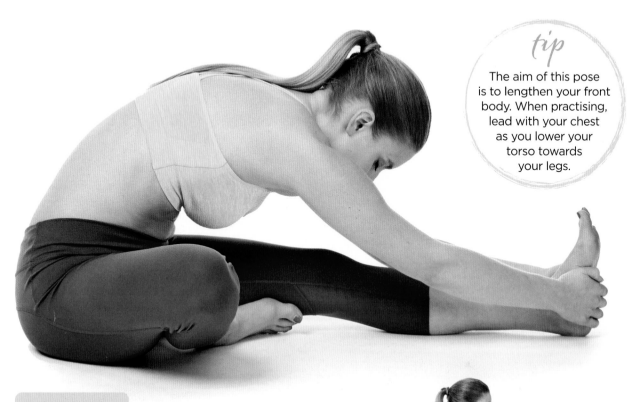

SITTING

HEAD TO KNEE POSE
Janu sirsasana

● From Staff pose (p50), fold your right leg in, so your heel touches your pubic bone and the sole rests on your inner thigh. Draw your left hip back and your right hip forwards to square your hips.
● Flex your left foot, spread your toes and reach through the ball of your foot. Place your hands either side of your left thigh and draw your navel to your spine.
● Inhale and root through your fingertips and sitting bones to lengthen your torso. Then, on an exhale, fold forwards from your hips, leading with your chest. Keep your spine long, core engaged and shoulder blades in and down. As you get lower, take your hands to your shin, ankle or sole of the foot.

● Inhale again, to lengthen, then exhale and fold a little further forwards. When you can go no further, release your head down towards your right knee.
● Breathe evenly and deeply for up to two minutes. Release to come up to sitting. Pause. Repeat on the other side.

GOOD FOR
✦ Improving circulation in your spine
✦ Strengthening your spine and legs
✦ Relieving tension in your lower back
✦ Quietening your mind

VARIATION
Place a strap around the ball of your front foot and hold one end in each hand. This will help you lower with a flat back while you build up your flexibility.

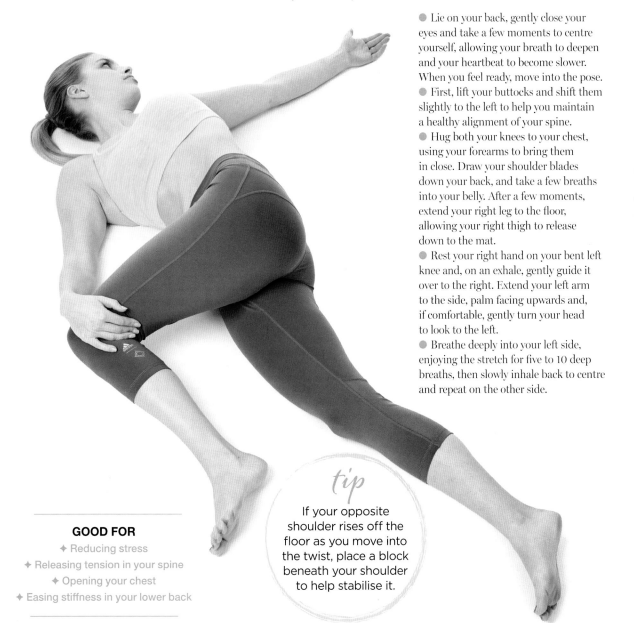

COOL DOWN/RELAXATION

RECLINING TWIST II
Supta parivartanasana II

- Lie on your back, gently close your eyes and take a few moments to centre yourself, allowing your breath to deepen and your heartbeat to become slower. When you feel ready, move into the pose.
- First, lift your buttocks and shift them slightly to the left to help you maintain a healthy alignment of your spine.
- Hug both your knees to your chest, using your forearms to bring them in close. Draw your shoulder blades down your back, and take a few breaths into your belly. After a few moments, extend your right leg to the floor, allowing your right thigh to release down to the mat.
- Rest your right hand on your bent left knee and, on an exhale, gently guide it over to the right. Extend your left arm to the side, palm facing upwards and, if comfortable, gently turn your head to look to the left.
- Breathe deeply into your left side, enjoying the stretch for five to 10 deep breaths, then slowly inhale back to centre and repeat on the other side.

tip

If your opposite shoulder rises off the floor as you move into the twist, place a block beneath your shoulder to help stabilise it.

GOOD FOR

✦ Reducing stress
✦ Releasing tension in your spine
✦ Opening your chest
✦ Easing stiffness in your lower back

THE SEQUENCE

This week we focus on grounding. If you have a solid foundation, your poses will be more stable and balanced

Time: 60 minutes

KEY POSE
Mountain pose

● Last week you tried Mountain pose (p29). Now you're familiar with its basic outline, it's time to look a bit deeper into how it's constructed. In the same way that the foundation of a building determines the strength and stability of the structure above ground, in yoga, the area of your body that touches the floor plays a key role in the quality of the final pose.

● In Mountain pose, your feet are your foundation. Take a moment to get into the pose then, using the image right, start fine-tuning your alignment, so you begin to feel the pose from the inside. A good way to begin is to sway gently from side to side, and back and forth, until you have a sense of the central position, where your weight is equally balanced between both feet and the front and back of your body.

● As you become familiar with the pose, you'll see how it forms the basis of many standing poses. Practise it whenever you have a spare moment, and notice the difference it makes to your posture and sense of being present in the moment.

CROWN
Let your crown lift towards the ceiling

NECK
Lengthen the back of your neck

SHOULDER BLADES
Release your shoulder blades down your spine

TAILBONE
Release your tailbone to the floor

ABDOMEN
Draw your navel to your spine

THIGHS
Rotate your upper thighs outwards

FEET
Press into the ground with the base of your big and little toes. Draw your ankles away from the midline to raise your inner arches

tip In your practice this week, notice where your attention is and bring your awareness to the part of the body that is touching the mat. Root into the earth beneath you, without thinking too much about what the pose 'should' look like. Return to the present, to your feet, feeling the pose from the inside.

ARRIVE/PREPARE

This week, give your attention to your feet, and imagine your out-breath travelling down your legs and through the soles of your feet

TAKE FIVE BREATHS IN EACH POSE UNLESS OTHERWISE STATED

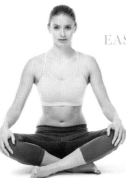

1 EASY POSE (p24)
Breathe into your belly for one to two minutes to quieten your mind

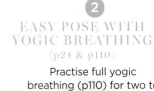

2 EASY POSE WITH YOGIC BREATHING (p24 & p110)
Practise full yogic breathing (p110) for two to three minutes, this time in Easy pose rather than lying on your back. You can place your hands on your lower belly, side ribs or chest as you breathe into that area of your body

WARM-UP

1 EASY POSE ONE ARM OVERHEAD (p24)
TORSO
Extend your side body

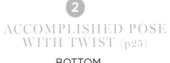

2 ACCOMPLISHED POSE WITH TWIST (p25)
BOTTOM
Keep both sitting bones connected to the ground

HANDS
Spread your fingers wide, middle finger pointing forwards

Repeat stages 4 and 5 on the other side

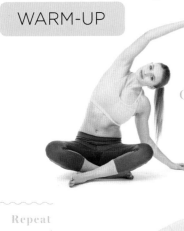

5 SIDE GATE (P45)
FOOT
Root through the outside edge of your back foot

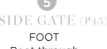

FEET
Keep your feet parallel and hip-width apart

3 CAT/COW (p27)
10 breaths

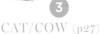

ARMS
Keep your elbows unlocked

4 TIGER (p44)
HANDS
Push the floor away to help lift your torso

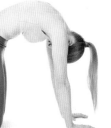

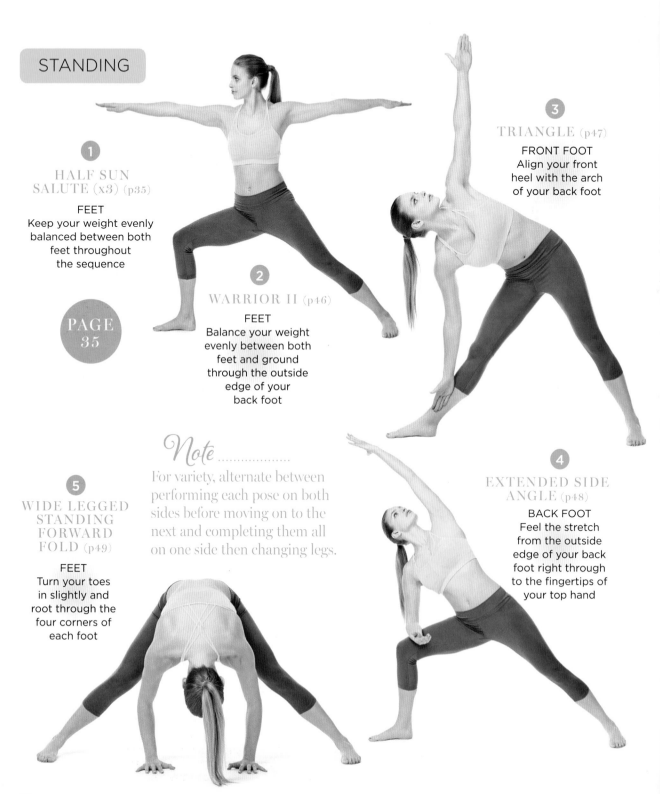

STANDING

1

HALF SUN SALUTE (x3) (p35)

FEET
Keep your weight evenly balanced between both feet throughout the sequence

PAGE 35

2

WARRIOR II (p46)

FEET
Balance your weight evenly between both feet and ground through the outside edge of your back foot

3

TRIANGLE (p47)

FRONT FOOT
Align your front heel with the arch of your back foot

Note ....
For variety, alternate between performing each pose on both sides before moving on to the next and completing them all on one side then changing legs.

4

EXTENDED SIDE ANGLE (p48)

BACK FOOT
Feel the stretch from the outside edge of your back foot right through to the fingertips of your top hand

5

WIDE LEGGED STANDING FORWARD FOLD (p49)

FEET
Turn your toes in slightly and root through the four corners of each foot

SITTING

1
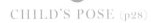
CHILD'S POSE (p28)

FEET, KNEES, FOREHEAD
Let your weight sink into the ground and be aware of the touch of the floor against your body

2
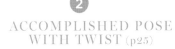
ACCOMPLISHED POSE WITH TWIST (p25)

SITTING BONES
Use your hands to separate the flesh of your sitting bones

3

STAFF POSE (p50)

FEET
Engage your feet as if you were in Mountain pose. Spread your toes, extend through the base of your big and little toes and lift the inner arches

Move with your breath

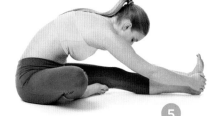

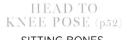
5
HEAD TO KNEE POSE (p52)

SITTING BONES
Make sure both sitting bones rest evenly on the ground

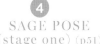

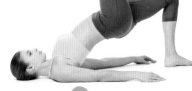
6
RAISED LEG BRIDGE (x2 each side) (p32)

FOOT
Keep your foot directly below your knee and root down to stablise the pose and keep your hips square

4
SAGE POSE (stage one) (p51)

FEET
Keep both feet active, the ankle of your straight leg flexed and your toes pointing to the ceiling

COOL DOWN/RELAXATION

1
KNEES TO CHEST (p33)

BACK
Allow your weight to sink into the floor

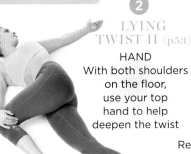

2
LYING TWIST II (p53)

HAND
With both shoulders on the floor, use your top hand to help deepen the twist

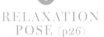

3
RELAXATION POSE (p26)

Rest for five minutes. Notice where your body is in contact with the floor and allow your muscles to soften and release on each out-breath

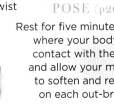

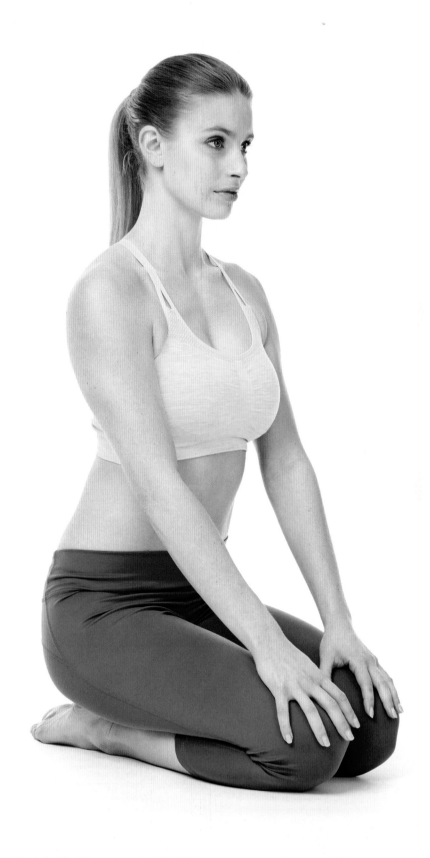

Week 3

Now that you've experienced what it's like to have a **strong foundation** to your poses, it's time to focus on your spine. The angle of your pelvis determines the position of **your spine** - tilt it forwards and your spine arches forwards, tip it backwards and your back will naturally round. This week you'll learn the three positions of the **pelvis used in yoga**, and put your learning into practice with this week's new poses and sequence on p68.

"IT IS THE JOB OF THE SPINE TO KEEP THE BRAIN ALERT. WHEN THE SPINE COLLAPSES, THE BRAIN COLLAPSES"

BKS Iyengar
Yoga teacher and author

THIS WEEK'S FOCUS

PELVIC ALIGNMENT

When standing with your pelvis in neutral, your spine should have four natural curves – two concave (neck and lower back) and two convex (mid back and sacrum). In yoga, the aim is to maintain these curves when standing

There are two other positions of your pelvis, which you've already encountered in the pose Cat/Cow (p27). **Cat tilt:** here your pelvis is tilted towards the back of your body. Your tail bone tucks under (if you scoop in your belly and draw your abdomen to your spine you'll feel it more strongly) and your lower back looses its natural arc. You use cat tilt at the beginning of Bridge pose (p32) to help you lengthen your spine before raising your hips. **Dog tilt:** this position is used at the beginning of many forward bends (for example Standing forward fold, p31) and helps keep your spine straight. Your tailbone is raised and tilted backwards and upwards. **Neutral pelvis:** imagine your pelvis as a bowl filled with water. If you were to tilt the top of your hips forwards (dog tilt) the water would flow over the front rim of the bowl; if you tuck your tailbone under and scoop in your belly (cat tilt), the water would trickle out the back of the bowl. When your pelvis is in neutral, the water stays

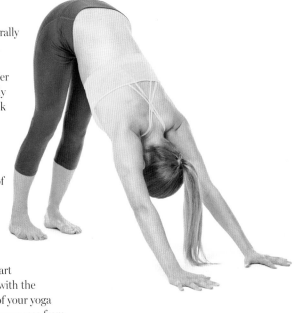

inside the bowl! As many people tend to stand naturally with their hips in dog tilt, over-arching their spine, remembering to tuck under your tailbone will naturally help bring your pelvis back in to neutral.

Your Week 3 yoga sessions

Over the first two weeks of your six-week beginner's guide we've shown you a handful of yoga's most iconic poses. Now is a good time to recap what you've learnt so far and start to become more familiar with the poses. This week, in one of your yoga sessions, choose two of three poses from the previous two weeks you would like to feel more confident with and work on them at a deeper level. Start to fine tune your alignment by observing your body and giving your attention to how the poses feel from the inside.

SUGGESTED PLAN

Session 1 (20 minutes) Recap your chosen poses from Weeks 1 and 2

Session 2 (20 minutes) Work on the new poses for Week 3

Session 3 (1 hour) Week 3 sequence

WEEK THREE

NEW POSES

✦ Puppy dog

✦ Hero

✦ Half dog

✦ Downward dog

✦ Cobra

✦ Locust prep

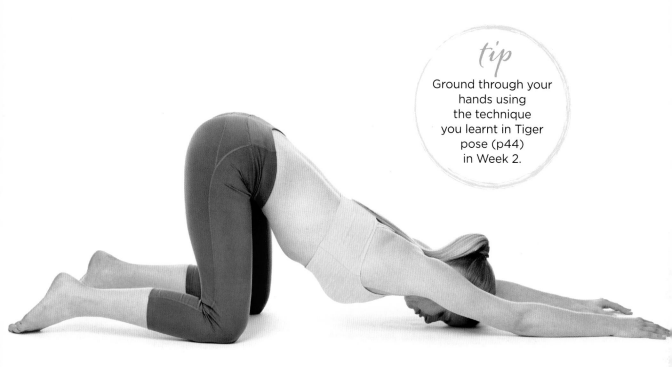

tip
Ground through your
hands using
the technique
you learnt in Tiger
pose (p44)
in Week 2.

WARM-UP

PUPPY DOG
Uttana shishosana

● Come onto all fours, with your shoulders directly above your wrists and your hips directly above your knees. Keep your shins and feet parallel and rest the tops of your toes on the floor, then walk your hands forwards a hand's-length or two.

● Inhale, then on an exhale, root your hands into the floor as you take your hips back slightly to lengthen your spine. Walk your hands forwards a few inches more, if needed, to keep your thighs vertical. Engage your arm muscles to keep them active and spread your fingertips, your middle finger pointing forwards.

● Allow your chest to softly release towards the floor as you lower your forehead to rest on the mat, block or a folded blanket. On your next inhalation, deepen into the stretch by reaching your hips back and up. Relax your neck and take five to 10 deep breaths into your back body.

● To come out of the pose, lift back up to all fours, then release into Child's pose (p28) and rest for a moment or two.

GOOD FOR
✦ Stretching your upper back, spine and shoulders
✦ Opening your chest
✦ Helping to release tension in your neck and shoulders

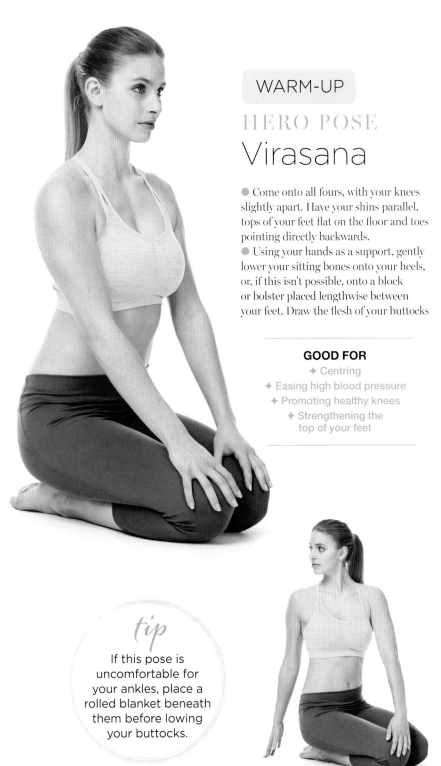

HERO POSE
Virasana

● Come onto all fours, with your knees slightly apart. Have your shins parallel, tops of your feet flat on the floor and toes pointing directly backwards.

● Using your hands as a support, gently lower your sitting bones onto your heels, or, if this isn't possible, onto a block or bolster placed lengthwise between your feet. Draw the flesh of your buttocks out to the sides, to allow your sitting bones to separate and your tailbone to release towards the floor.

● Lift up through your spine, maintaining its vertical alignment and take your front ribs slightly in towards your back.

● Draw your shoulder blades downwards and let your head balance evenly and lightly on the top of your spine. Lengthen the back of your neck and lift up through your crown.

● Rest your hands on your thighs, palms up or down, whichever feels most comfortable. If you like, gently close your eyes.

● Breathe fully and deeply for up to one minute, letting your weight sink deeper on the exhale, a gentle expansion on the inhale.

GOOD FOR
✦ Centring
✦ Easing high blood pressure
✦ Promoting healthy knees
✦ Strengthening the top of your feet

VARIATION
Hero twist
Place your right hand on the floor behind your right buttock, fingers pointing back and down or, if possible, place your palm on the floor, and rest your left palm on your right knee. Inhale as you root through your sitting bones to lift your spine out of your pelvis. On an exhale, slowly rotate your spine to the right, moving in a spiral from your waist initially, then your upper body. Inhale, lengthen through the crown of your head, and exhale further into the twist. If comfortable for your neck, turn your head to look over your right shoulder. Inhale back to centre and repeat on the other side.

tip
If this pose is uncomfortable for your ankles, place a rolled blanket beneath them before lowing your buttocks.

STANDING

HALF DOG
Ardha adho mukha svanasana

tip

Really work at reaching back with your tailbone. This is the same movement you'll be doing in Downward dog (p65).

● Stand with your feet hip-distance apart two to three feet from a wall and rest your palms on its surface at a comfortable height. Slowly walk your hands down the wall, adjusting your feet if you need so that you can take your arms and torso parallel to the floor.

● Root through your feet, spread your toes and ground through the base of your big and little toes. Draw your ankles apart to lift your arches and bend your knees as much as is needed to maintain a flat back.

● With your fingers spread and hands rooting into the wall, lightly engage your core to support your lower back, draw your shoulder blades down your spine to create space around your shoulders and lengthen your neck, keeping it in line with your spine. As you root into the wall with your hands, extend your tailbone towards the opposite wall and enjoy the feeling of stretching out your spine. Take five to 10 breaths, and then release on an exhale.

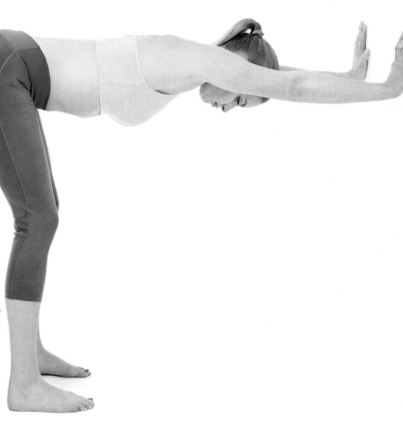

GOOD FOR
✦ Extending your spine
✦ Strengthening your arms
✦ Stretching your hamstrings
✦ Preparing for Downward dog

STANDING

DOWNWARD DOG
Adho mukha svanasana

● Start on all fours, knees beneath your hips, and place your hands a palm's-length in front of your shoulders, shoulder-width apart, fingers spread and middle finger pointing forwards.
● Root through the base of your thumbs and index fingers, tuck under your toes and raise your knees off the mat, taking your tailbone back and up into dog tilt to lengthen your spine (A).
● Keeping your knees bent, imagine you are pushing the mat away from you with your hands as you extend your spine.

Draw your shoulder blades down your back as you rotate your upper arms externally, then lower your front ribs towards your thighs and release your neck.
● 'Walk the dog' by gently taking one heel and then the other towards the mat (B), stretching out your hamstrings in a walking motion.
● Spread your toes and lower both heels towards the mat. Check your weight is evenly distributed through each foot and your inner arches are lifted. Don't worry

if your heels don't reach the ground, this will become easier over time.
● Take five deep breaths then exhale and lower into Child's pose (p28).

GOOD FOR
✦ Insomnia
✦ Fatigue
✦ Calming your nervous system
✦ Easing palpitations

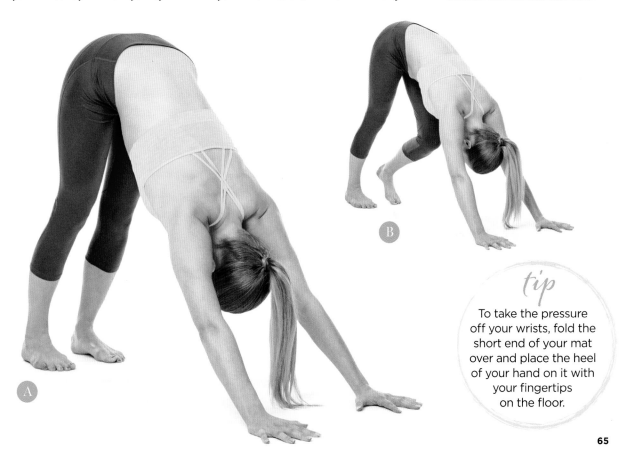

A

B

tip

To take the pressure off your wrists, fold the short end of your mat over and place the heel of your hand on it with your fingertips on the floor.

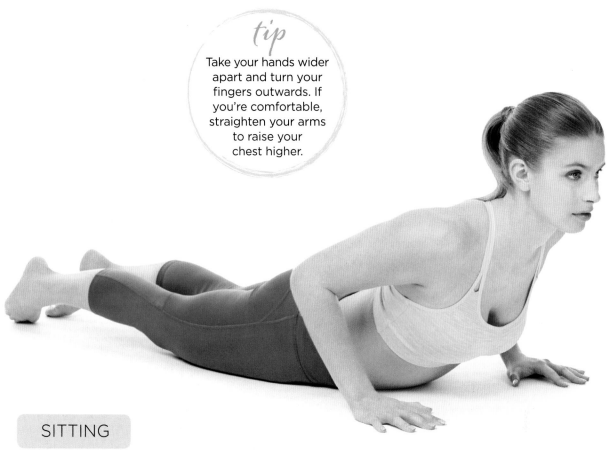

tip

Take your hands wider apart and turn your fingers outwards. If you're comfortable, straighten your arms to raise your chest higher.

SITTING

COBRA
Bhujangasana

● Lie on your stomach, feet hip–distance apart, legs and ankles straight and toes spread. Place your hands beneath your shoulders, palms down, fingers spread, middle fingers pointing forwards. Root through the base of your thumbs and index fingers.

● Draw your elbows together and rotate your shoulders up, back and down to create space in your neck, then release your shoulder blades down your back. Engage your abdomen and root through your pelvic bone.

● Inhale, and raise your head and shoulders as far as is comfortable by drawing the back of your neck upwards, keeping your eyes looking down. Exhale.

● On an inhale, ground through your hands and curl your spine further forwards and up. Lengthen your spine evenly without compressing the back of your neck or lumbar spine. Lift your head last and gaze on the floor a few feet in front of you.

● Breathe normally for three to five breaths. Slowly and controlled, exhale as you lower your body to the floor one vertebra at a time and rest your head on one side.

GOOD FOR

✦ Strengthening your spine; toning your spinal nerves

✦ Easing tension in your back, shoulders and neck

✦ Helping to relieve stress and fatigue

✦ Opening your heart and lungs

LOCUST PREP

Salabasana prep

● Lie on your tummy, with your forehead resting on the mat and arms at your sides, palms facing upwards. Take a few breaths to centre yourself. When you feel ready, turn your big toes towards each other to rotate your thighs inwards.

● On an inhale, draw your navel to your spine and lift your legs, stretching your legs right through to your pointed toes (A). Take up to five breaths, then exhale to release, and repeat twice more.

● On your next inhale, draw your navel to your spine, lengthen the back of your neck and raise your head, chest and arms away from the mat. Press your arms up against an imagined weight and bring your shoulder blades in towards your back. Gaze softly forwards (B). After five breaths, exhale to release, then repeat twice more.

● Turn to page 99 to see the full pose.

tip

Practising Locust in stages will help to strengthen your muscles in preparation for the full pose. Gradually increase how long you hold the pose for.

GOOD FOR

✦ Strengthening your back, buttocks, arms and legs

✦ Opening your shoulders, chest, belly and thighs

✦ Improving your posture

✦ Relieving stress

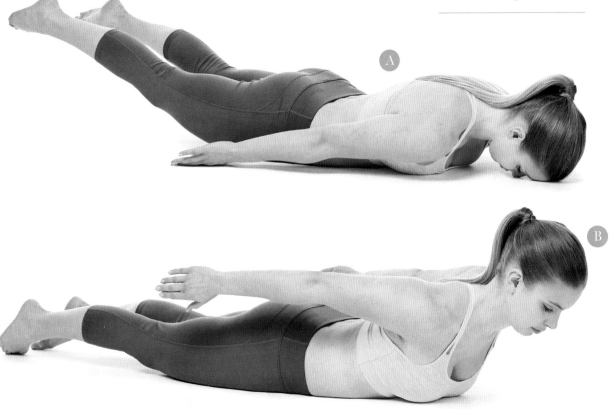

THE SEQUENCE

This week we focus on the position of the pelvis to understand
how it relates to the alignment of the spine

Time: 60 minutes

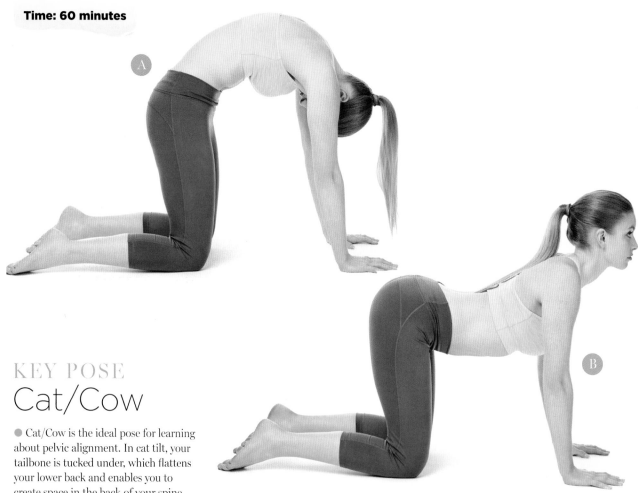

KEY POSE
Cat/Cow

● Cat/Cow is the ideal pose for learning
about pelvic alignment. In cat tilt, your
tailbone is tucked under, which flattens
your lower back and enables you to
create space in the back of your spine
(A). By lifting your tailbone to the
sky you come into dog tilt, your lower
back curves more deeply and you're
able to lengthen your spine more fully
(B). Practise moving between these two
poses slowly and mindfully, one vertebra
at a time and in time with your breath,
and allow your body to absorb the
sensation of each position.

tip In all your poses
this week, give
attention to your
hips. Explore
how adjusting your pelvis
changes your overall
experience of the pose.

ARRIVE/PREPARE

TAKE FIVE BREATHS IN EACH POSE UNLESS OTHERWISE STATED

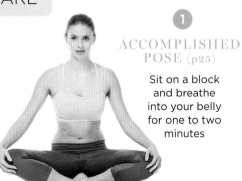

①

ACCOMPLISHED POSE (p25)

Sit on a block and breathe into your belly for one to two minutes

Note ....
Lightly draw your navel to your spine to support your lower back

WARM-UP

HIPS
Pause for a moment in dog tilt

②

HERO TWIST (p63)

PELVIS
Before you twist, take your hips into dog and cat tilt and notice the effect on your spine

①

CAT/COW (p68)

10 breaths

HIPS
Pause for a moment in cat tilt

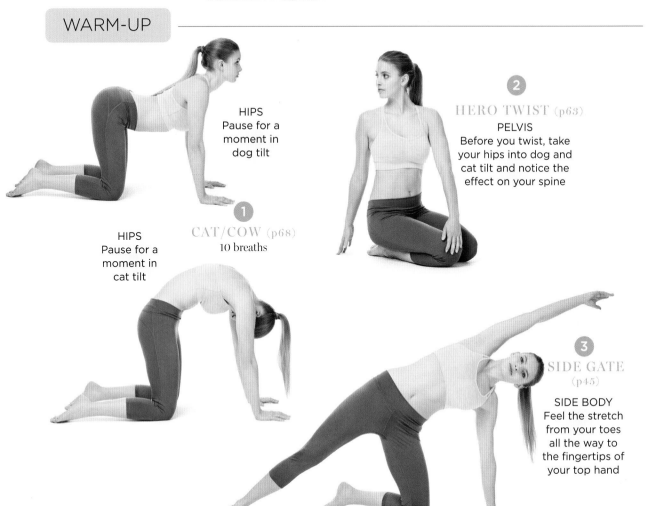

③

SIDE GATE (p45)

SIDE BODY
Feel the stretch from your toes all the way to the fingertips of your top hand

STANDING

1

MOUNTAIN
POSE (p29)

FEET
Be still for
a moment,
grounding through
your feet as in last
week's lesson

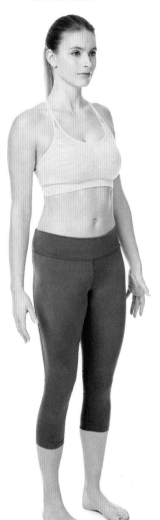

2

HALF SUN
SALUTE (x3)(p35)

PELVIS
Fold forwards with
a flat back, hips
in dog tilt. Uncurl
your spine to
return to standing,
hips in cat tilt

PAGE
35

Remember to use
pada bandha to
ground through
your feet and hasta
bandha to root
through your hands

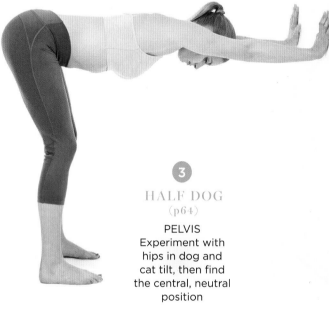

3

HALF DOG
(p64)

PELVIS
Experiment with
hips in dog and
cat tilt, then find
the central, neutral
position

4

DOWNWARD
DOG (p65)

BACK BODY
Feel the stretch from
your hands (in hasta
bandha) all the way
to your tailbone,
which reaches up and
back (in dog tilt)

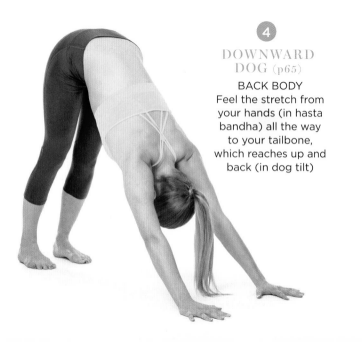

SITTING

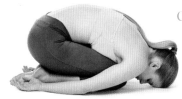

1

CHILD'S POSE (p28)

LOWER BACK
Rest for a moment
or two as you
breathe into your
back body

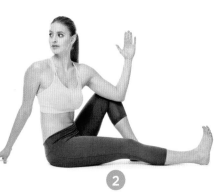

2

SAGE POSE (stage two) (p51)

LOWER BACK
If your spine rounds (ie cat tilt
hips), sit on a block to bring
your pelvis into neutral

6

BRIDGE (x2) (p32)

PELVIS
Bring your hips into cat tilt to
raise your hips, dog tilt at the top
of the move, then shift your hips
back into cat tilt as you uncurl
your spine to lower to the floor

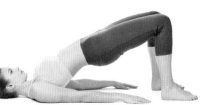

3

HEAD TO KNEE POSE (p52)

PELVIS
Fold forwards with a
flat back initially, hips
in dog tilt, then use cat
tilt as your torso lowers
towards your thighs

5

LOCUST PREP (p67)

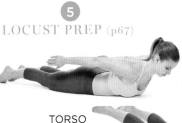

UPPER BACK
Bring your shoulder
blades in towards
your back

4

COBRA (p66)

HIPS
Press your
pubic bone
into the mat

TORSO
Draw your
navel to
your spine

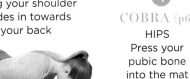

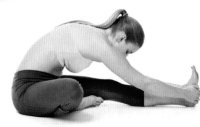

COOL DOWN/RELAXATION

1

KNEES TO CHEST (p33)

BACK
Is your pelvis in
dog tilt or cat tilt?

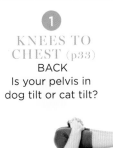

2

LYING TWIST II (p53)

HIPS
Shift your hips to
the right before
twisting to the left,
and vice versa

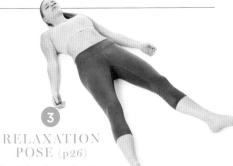

3

RELAXATION POSE (p26)

Rest for five minutes
breathing naturally and
allowing your muscles
to soften and sink
into the floor

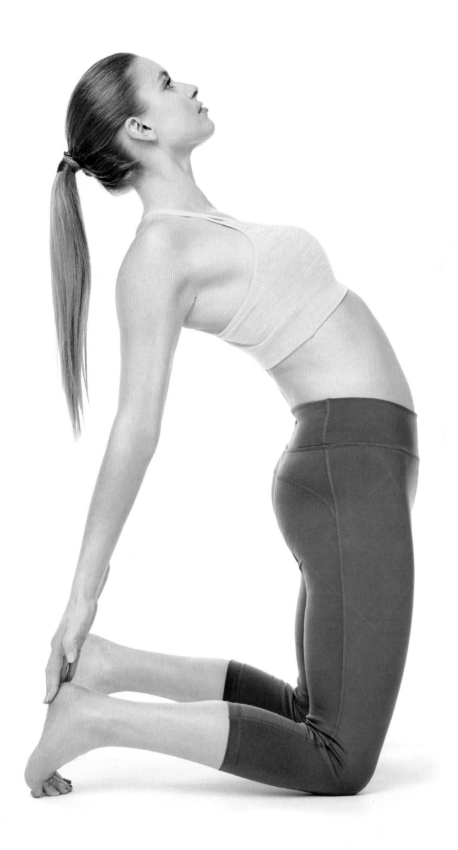

Week 4

Well done for reaching the **half-way point** in your six-week introduction to yoga! By now you're likely to be enjoying the benefits of **increased flexibility**, greater strength and a more peaceful mind. This week, we'll work on learning to **lengthen the spine** to energise not just your poses, but your life off the mat too. You'll also be able to integrate all you've learnt so far - yogic breathing, **grounding through your feet** and hands and the correct position of your pelvis – in a Beginner's sun salute on p86.

" EXERCISE IS LIKE PROSE,

WHEREAS YOGA IS THE POETRY

OF MOVEMENT. ONCE YOU

UNDERSTAND THE GRAMMAR OF

YOGA; YOU CAN WRITE YOUR

OWN POETRY "

Amit Ray
Author, philosopher and
spiritual master

INTEGRATION OF BREATH, FOUNDATION & SPINE

When these elements work together, a transformation occurs in your yoga practice. The poses feel more dynamic, you experience a sense of inner and outer strength, and a nourishing quality accompanies each breath you take

The Beginner's sun salute (p86) is ideal for learning to integrate your practice in this way, especially when you work in a slow, mindful manner. The repeated flexion and extension of your back in Sun salutes is also very beneficial for your spine – which needs regular exercise to maintain its flexibility. Your spinal discs also need to be well hydrated. These spongy structures protect and separate the vertebrae and help absorb shock but, to do their job properly, they need to be hydrated. By rhythmically compressing and releasing, as happens in a Sun salute, your discs attract the water they need.

If you want to continue working with integration when you're not on your yoga mat, you might like to try mindful walking. As you walk about in your daily life, from time to time, take your attention to the soles of your feet. Notice the subtly graded sensations you experience as you transition your weight from your heels to the balls of your feet, and from one foot to the other.

On other occasions, tune in to your breath, observing the rise and fall of your chest or abdomen. Another time, be aware of your pelvis and spine – are your shoulders relaxed? Are they balanced over your pelvis? Finally, when you are walking some distance, see if you can broaden your attention to take in all three.

Your Week 4 yoga sessions

By now you'll be starting to get a sense of which poses you feel comfortable with and which are more of a challenge. If you're designing your own sessions, you can begin to be a little more sophisticated, so aim to include a couple of warm-ups before you start your main practice, and include both standing and sitting postures before you finish with Relaxation pose (p26).

If you're short on time, a few rounds of Half (p35) and then Beginner's sun salute are a great way to incorporate yoga into your life on a daily basis.

WEEK FOUR

NEW POSES
✦ Reclining butterfly
✦ Happy baby
✦ Reclining hand-to-toe
✦ Hero with cow face arms
✦ Crescent prep
✦ Standing forward fold with shoulder stretch
✦ High lunge
✦ Pyramid
✦ Camel
✦ Reclining wide angle pose

NEW SEQUENCE
✦ Beginner's sun salute

SUGGESTED PLAN

Session 1 (25 minutes) Chose 2 or 3 warm-ups, Beginner's sun salute and seated poses

Session 2 (25 minutes) The remaining warm-ups, Beginner's sun salute and standing poses

Session 3 (1 hour) Week 4 sequence

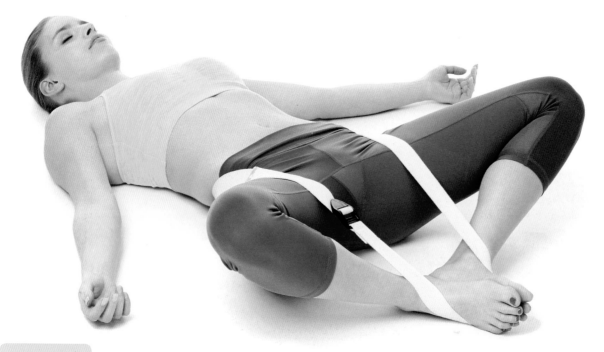

ARRIVE

RECLINING BUTTERFLY

Supta baddha konasana

● Sit on your mat and bring the soles of your feet together. Loop a strap around your back, over your thighs and around your feet and adjust to fit, making sure the buckle doesn't press into your legs. Gently lower back onto your forearms, then continue lowering until your back is flat on the mat, using your arms to support you.

● Let your knees gently fall out to the sides to create a diamond shape with your legs. Place your arms out to the sides, palms facing up.

● Make any minor adjustments you need, so there is no strain on any part of your body. If your neck is uncomfortable, place a thin blanket beneath your head.

● Gently close your eyes, connect to your breath and surrender your weight to the earth. Rest here for as long as is comfortable – up to 10 minutes. Then gently bring your knees together, loosen the strap, shift your bottom to the left, let your knees fall to your right, and slowly roll your body over to the right. Pause here for a moment, before using your hands to gently bring you up to sitting.

tip

If you feel your hips are tight and you don't have a strap, place a block or cushion underneath each knee.

GOOD FOR

✦ Calming your nervous system

✦ Regulating blood pressure

✦ Opening your hips and heart area

WARM-UP

WARM-UP

HAPPY BABY
Ananda balasana

● Lie on your back and take a moment to centre yourself. Take three deep breaths, allowing your weight to sink into the floor as you exhale.

● When you feel ready, bend your knees deeply, take hold of your big toes with the index finger of each hand and open your knees, allowing them to release down towards your armpits.

● Flex your ankles, soles facing the ceiling, and bring your calves as near to vertical as possible. Feel the stretch in your groins and a deep release in your lower back.

● Tuck in your chin to lengthen your neck, and draw your shoulders down your spine to create space around your neck. Reach your tailbone forwards to lengthen your spine.

● Stay here for 10-20 slow deep breaths, then rock gently from side to side before releasing your feet to the floor.

GOOD FOR
✦ Relieving stress
✦ Opening your inner and outer thighs
✦ Easing lower back tension

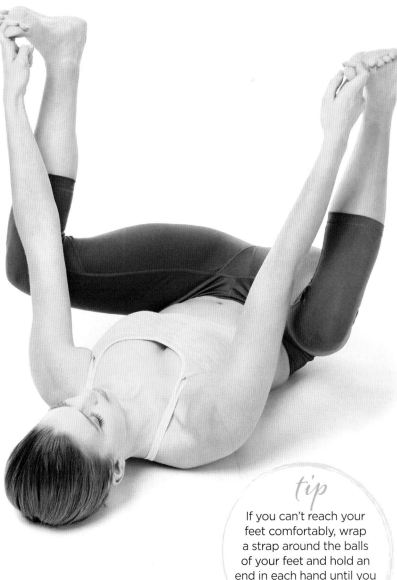

tip

If you can't reach your feet comfortably, wrap a strap around the balls of your feet and hold an end in each hand until you become more flexible and no longer need it.

WARM-UP

RECLINING HAND-TO-TOE POSE
Supta padangusthasana

● Lie on your back, knees bent and feet flat on the floor close to your buttocks. Slowly extend your right leg, flex your ankle, spread the toes of your right foot, extending your big and little toes away from you, making sure your big toe is pointing towards the ceiling. Reach through the heel and the ball of your right foot.

● Bend your left knee in to your chest and wrap a yoga strap around the ball of your foot, holding both ends of the strap in your left hand.

● Slowly extend your left leg, keeping your ankle flexed and reaching through your left heel, taking it as close to vertical as is comfortable.

● Lightly engage your core, draw your shoulders down your spine and keep both legs active. Take five to 10 deep breaths, walking your hands up the strap as the pose becomes more comfortable and your flexibility increases.

● When you feel ready, gently lower your leg on an exhale, and repeat on the other side.

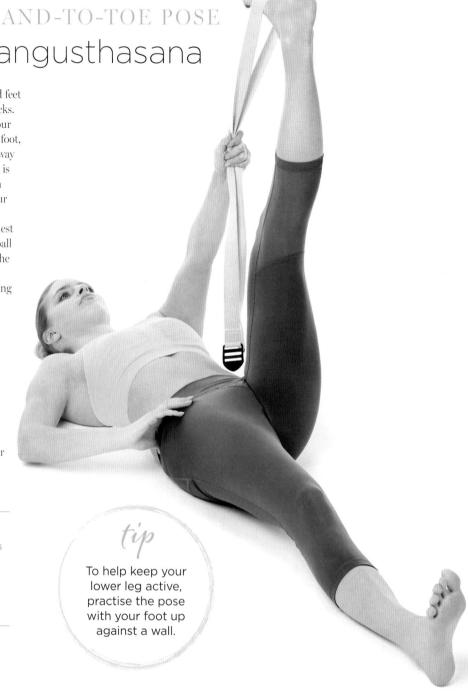

GOOD FOR

✦ Stretching your hamstrings and calves

✦ Opening your hips

✦ Relieving backache

✦ Strengthening your knees

tip

To help keep your lower leg active, practise the pose with your foot up against a wall.

HERO WITH COW FACE ARMS
Virasana with gumukasna arms

● Spend a few moments in Hero pose (p63) to still your mind then, when you feel ready, on an inhale, take your right arm out to the side, palm facing the ceiling. As you exhale, bring your arm behind your back, forearm on your lower back and palm facing away from you. Lift your hand to bring it towards the centre of your shoulder blades, palm still facing backwards.

● On you next inhale, extend your left arm in front of you and overhead, with your palm facing the back of the room. As you exhale, bend your left elbow and reach down for your right hand, clasping your fingers together if possible.

● Lift your left elbow, and allow your right elbow to release towards the floor. Draw your shoulders down your spine and lift your chest. Take five breaths then release and repeat on the other side.

GOOD FOR
✦ Opening your chest
✦ Stretching your shoulders, triceps and chest
✦ Easing backache
✦ Reducing tiredness

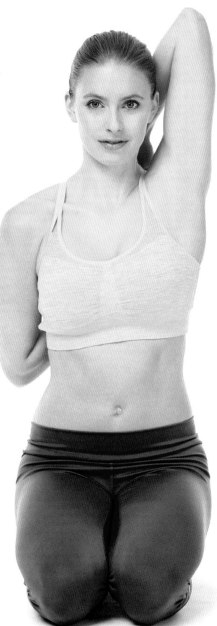

tip

Practise this pose using a strap between your hands. Walk your hands closer together as your flexibility increases.

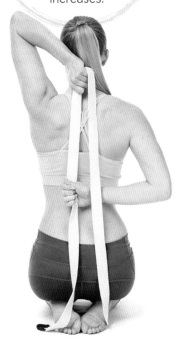

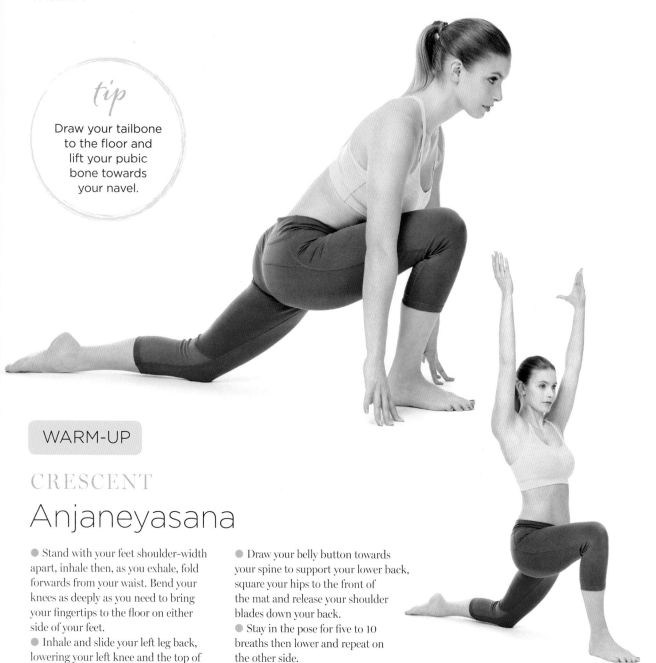

tip

Draw your tailbone to the floor and lift your pubic bone towards your navel.

WARM-UP

CRESCENT
Anjaneyasana

● Stand with your feet shoulder-width apart, inhale then, as you exhale, fold forwards from your waist. Bend your knees as deeply as you need to bring your fingertips to the floor on either side of your feet.

● Inhale and slide your left leg back, lowering your left knee and the top of your left foot onto the floor. Exhale. Spread the toes of your right foot, pressing down through your big and little toes. Draw your ankle out to the side to lift your inner arch.

● Square your hips to the front of the mat, and breath deeply here for a few moments, then inhale and bring both hands to rest on your right knee.

● Draw your belly button towards your spine to support your lower back, square your hips to the front of the mat and release your shoulder blades down your back.

● Stay in the pose for five to 10 breaths then lower and repeat on the other side.

GOOD FOR

✦ Balancing your nervous system

✦ Energising without overstimulating

✦ Helping sciatica

VARIATION
Full pose
When you feel strong in the pose, with your hands on the floor, on an inhale draw your abdomen to your spine and raise your torso, taking your hands overhead, palms facing. Take five deep breaths then release on an exhale.

STANDING FORWARD FOLD (SHOULDER STRETCH)

Uttanasana

● Place your feet shoulder-width apart, inner edges parallel. Balance your weight evenly over each foot, spread your toes and root through the base of your big and little toes. Lift your inner arches by drawing your ankles away from each other.

● Interlace your fingers behind your back and draw your shoulder blades together to take your shoulders down and back. On an inhale, lengthen your spine, then as you exhale, fold forwards with your hips in dog tilt, raising your hands back and up as you do so. Allow your back to round as you get lower, your hips coming into cat tilt, and release your head towards the floor. Take a few breaths here, then gently uncurl to come back up to standing.

GOOD FOR

✦ Opening your chest and shoulders
✦ Strengthening your back
✦ Calming
✦ Refreshing your mind

tip

You can do the pose with your arms folded behind your back, hands to elbows. Remember to raise your elbows as you fold towards the floor.

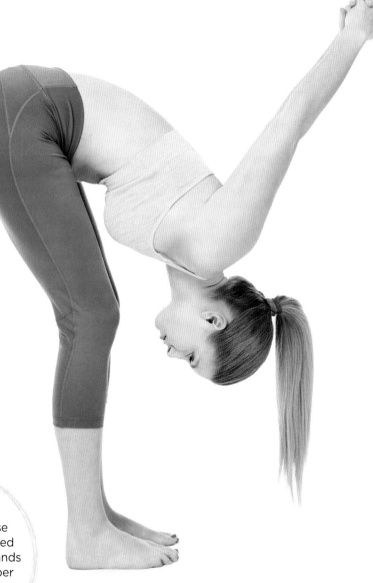

STANDING

HIGH LUNGE
Alanasana

● Stand with your feet hip-width apart, inner edges parallel, and fold forwards to place your hands either side of your feet. Take a large step straight back with your left leg to rest on the ball of your foot. Straighten your leg and extend through your back heel. Your right knee is directly over your right ankle, aligned with your middle toes.

● Ground through your feet, engage your core and, on an inhale, rise up to bring your torso to vertical, resting your hands on your hips.

● Pause here for a moment as you check that your hips are square to the front of your mat, lengthen your spine out of your pelvis and draw your shoulder blades down your spine.

● On your next inhale, sweep your arms out to the sides and overhead.

● Breathe evenly into your belly for five deep breaths, then release your arms on an exhale, bring your hands either side of your front foot, step your back foot forwards and repeat on the other side.

GOOD FOR

✦ Strengthening your legs
✦ Releasing tension in your hips
✦ Aiding balance

tip

If you find it difficult to square your hips to the front, take your back foot slightly wider.

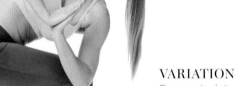

VARIATION
Prayer twist

From high lunge, with your hands in prayer position in front of your heart, inhale then, as you exhale, twist your spine to the right, and rest your left elbow on the outside of your right knee. Take a couple of breaths, then release on an exhale and repeat on the other side.

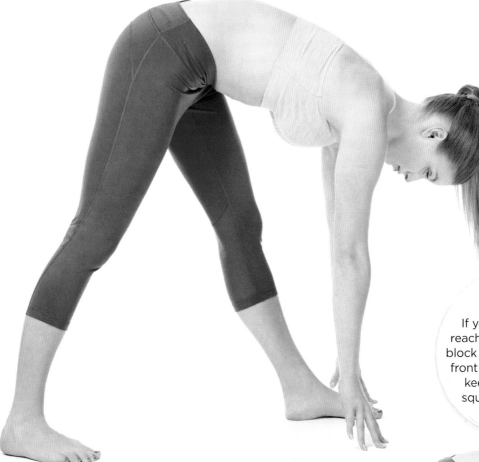

tip

If your hands don't reach the floor, place a block either side of your front foot and work on keeping your hips square to the front of your mat.

STANDING

PYRAMID

Parsvottanasana

● With your feet parallel and hip-width apart, take a large step back with your right leg, turning your toes out 45 degrees. Spread your toes wide, ground through the big and little toes of both feet and lift your inner arches by drawing your ankles apart.

● Place your hands on your hips, bringing your right hip forwards and your left hip back to square your pelvis, then draw your inner thighs towards each other.

● Inhale and root into the ground as you lengthen your spine then, on an exhale, begin to fold forwards, keeping your spine flat.

● On your next inhale, extend and lengthen your spine again, then gently release on an exhale to fold forwards even more. Let your back curve naturally as you lower yourself and take your hands to the floor.

● Rest in the pose for five to 10 breaths, breathing evenly. When you feel ready, root through your feet, engage your core and inhale to return to standing. Exhale to step your feet together, pause for a moment, then repeat on the other side.

GOOD FOR
✦ Increasing blood flow to your head
✦ Calming your mind
✦ Aiding deep breathing
✦ Developing balance

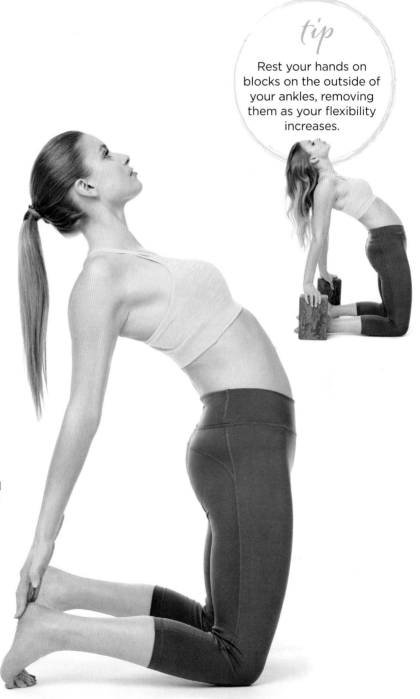

SITTING

CAMEL
Ustrasana

● Kneel with your thighs hip-width apart, toes tucked under. Inhale, lengthen your spine out of your pelvis and circle your right arm overhead and rest it on your right heel. Exhale. Take a few breaths to become accustomed to the stretch.

● On your next inhale, repeat the same move with your left hand. Keep your eyes looking ahead so that you don't strain your neck. Exhale.

● As you inhale, lift your sternum gently upwards, opening your chest and shoulders. Release your tailbone towards the floor to feel the stretch in your quads and core.

● Maintain the length in your neck, and tuck your chin in slightly. Take five to 10 deep breaths, then release on an exhale, using your core muscles to help you come to an upright position. Rest for a few moments in Child's pose (p28).

GOOD FOR
✦ Boosting energy
✦ Deep chest and heart opener
✦ Strengthening your thighs
✦ Opening your hip flexors

RECLINING WIDE ANGLE POSE
Supta upavista konasana

● Place the short end of your mat against a wall, then sit sideways on the mat, close to the wall. Bend your knees and have your feet flat on the floor.

● Resting your palms on the floor behind you, fingertips pointing forwards, use your hands to help you roll onto your back as you simultaneously swing your legs up the wall and rotate your torso so you're lying on the centre of your mat. Take your legs as wide apart as is comfortable.

● Adjust your position if needed so your lower back rests comfortably on the mat, and release your arms by your sides, palms facing upwards.

● Stay in the pose for up to five minutes, allowing your breath to settle and your muscles to become heavy.

● To come out, bring your knees to your chest, resting here for a few breaths before gently rolling over to your right and using your hands to help you come up to sitting.

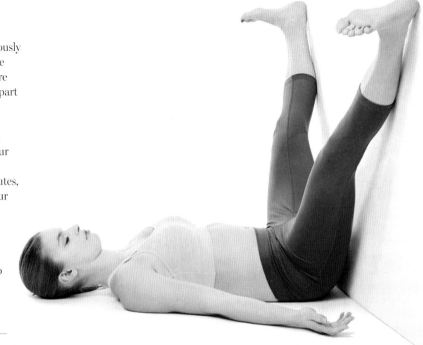

GOOD FOR
✦ Reducing fatigue in your legs
✦ Quietening your mind
✦ Improving your circulation

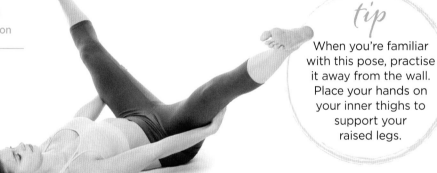

tip
When you're familiar with this pose, practise it away from the wall. Place your hands on your inner thighs to support your raised legs.

Beginner's surya namaskar

Sun salutes are a great way to prepare your body for the main poses in your yoga session

● On the first round, take three to five breaths in each pose to let you feel confident with your alignment and allow your body to acclimatise to the pose. Repeat the round once or twice more, following the breathing pattern below as you become familiar with the sequence.

1 Mountain pose prayer hands (p29) Inhale, root through your feet then take your arms out to the sides and overhead to...

2 Extended mountain pose (p30) Exhale and take your arms to the sides and down to...

3 Standing forward fold (p31) Inhale to...

4 Half standing forward fold (p31) Exhale as you step your right leg back to...

5 Crescent (p80) Inhale. Step your left leg back to...

6 Downward dog (p65) Exhale and step your right leg forward to...

7 Crescent (p80) Exhale and step your left foot forward to...

8 Standing forward fold (p31) Inhale, taking your arms out to the side and overhead to...

9 Extended mountain pose (p30) Exhale your arms out to the side and to prayer, back to...

10 Mountain pose prayer hands (p29) Repeat, leading with your left leg. This is one round.

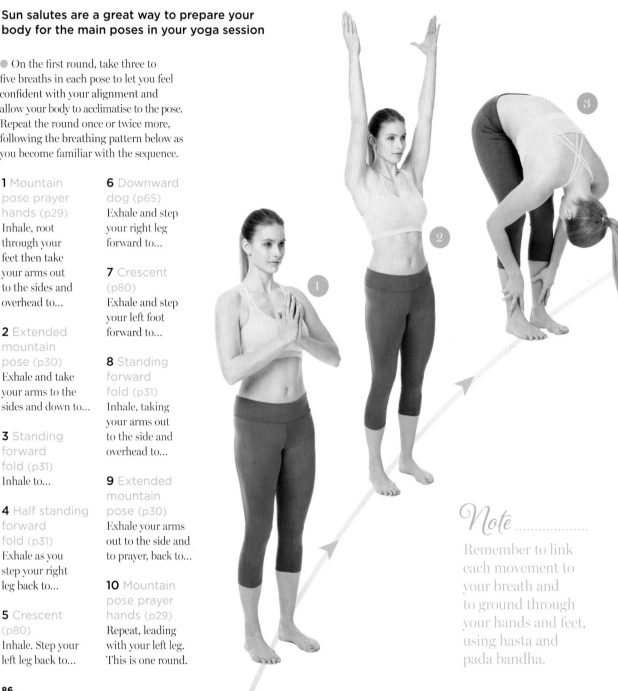

Note ....
Remember to link each movement to your breath and to ground through your hands and feet, using hasta and pada bandha.

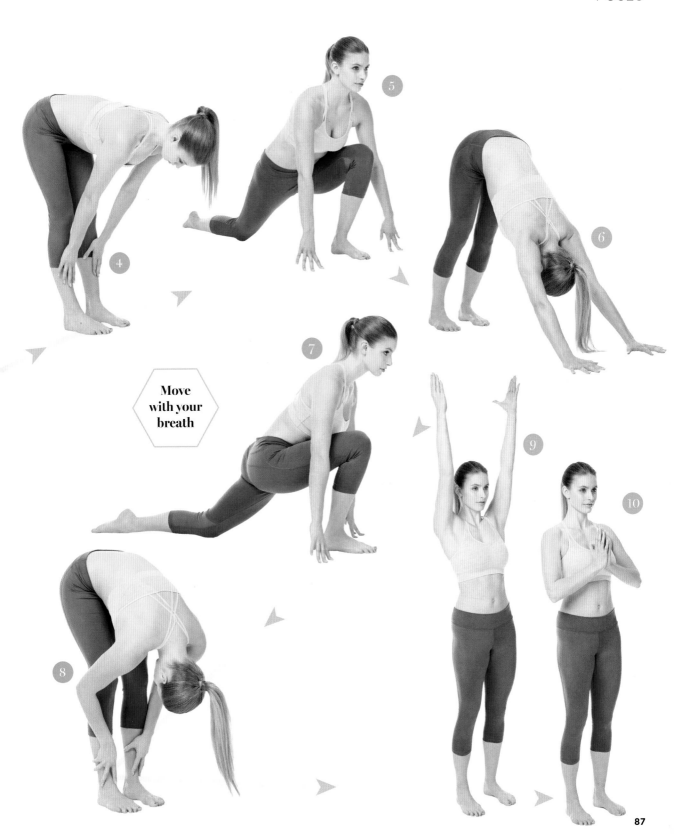

Move with your breath

THE SEQUENCE

This week we bring together the elements of breath, foundation and spine and learn how to integrate them in your practice

Time: 60 minutes

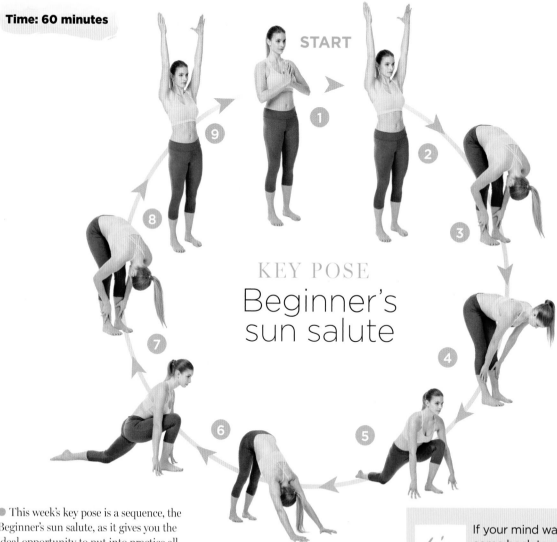

START

KEY POSE

Beginner's sun salute

● This week's key pose is a sequence, the Beginner's sun salute, as it gives you the ideal opportunity to put into practice all you have learnt so far. Using the previous two pages (p86-87), take your time to become familiar with the order of the poses and the breathing pattern before you do this week's sequence. The simplest way to remember is that you breathe in when you open your chest or bend backwards, and you breathe out as you close your chest or fold forwards. And remember to use pada bandha to ground through your feet and hasta bandha to root through your hands.

tip If your mind wanders, come back to your breath. Take deep breaths into your belly, let your mind settle and your body release into the ground. This will help you relax.

ARRIVE/PREPARE

TAKE FIVE BREATHS IN EACH POSE UNLESS OTHERWISE STATED

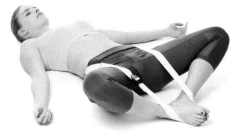

1

RECLINING BUTTERFLY (p76)

CHEST
Breathe normally for a minute or two before practising yogic breathing (p36) for five minutes

Move with your breath

WARM-UP

1

HAPPY BABY (p77)

HIPS
Reach your tailbone forwards to create length in your spine

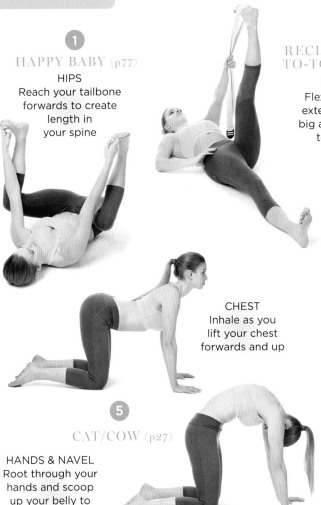

2

RECLINING HAND-TO-TOE POSE I (p78)

RIGHT FOOT
Flex your ankle and extend through your big and little toes, big toe pointing to the ceiling

When you have settled into a pose, try closing your eyes for a moment or two to get a sense of how the pose feels internally

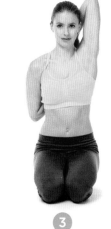

3

HERO POSE WITH COW FACE ARMS (p79)

UPPER BODY
Draw your shoulders down your spine and lift your chest

CHEST
Inhale as you lift your chest forwards and up

5

CAT/COW (p27)

HANDS & NAVEL
Root through your hands and scoop up your belly to lift your spine

4

CRESCENT (p80)

PELVIS
Square your hips to the front of the mat

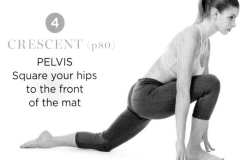

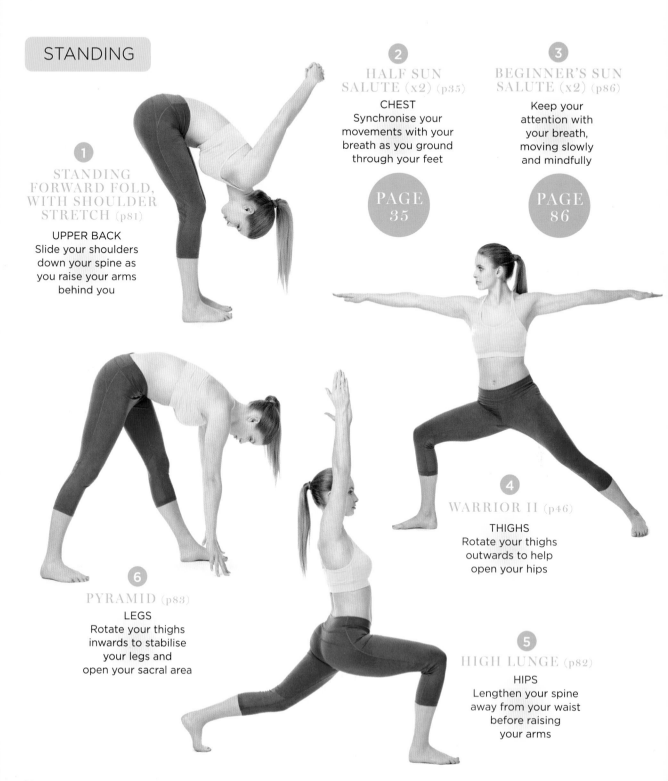

STANDING

1

STANDING
FORWARD FOLD,
WITH SHOULDER
STRETCH (p81)

UPPER BACK
Slide your shoulders
down your spine as
you raise your arms
behind you

2

HALF SUN
SALUTE (x2) (p35)

CHEST
Synchronise your
movements with your
breath as you ground
through your feet

PAGE
35

3

BEGINNER'S SUN
SALUTE (x2) (p86)

Keep your
attention with
your breath,
moving slowly
and mindfully

PAGE
86

4

WARRIOR II (p46)

THIGHS
Rotate your thighs
outwards to help
open your hips

6

PYRAMID (p83)

LEGS
Rotate your thighs
inwards to stabilise
your legs and
open your sacral area

5

HIGH LUNGE (p82)

HIPS
Lengthen your spine
away from your waist
before raising
your arms

SITTING

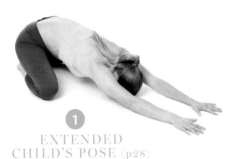

② CAMEL (p84)

BOTTOM
Release your
tailbone to the
floor to feel the
stretch in your
quads and core

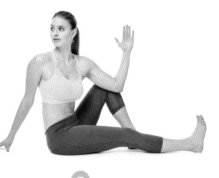

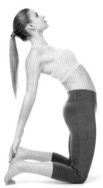

① EXTENDED CHILD'S POSE (p28)

BOTTOM
Release your sitting
bone to your heels
as you stretch
through to your
fingertips

③ SAGE POSE (stage two) (p51)

LOWER BACK
If your spine rounds
(ie cat tilt hips),
sit on a block to
bring your pelvis
into neutral

④ HEAD TO KNEE POSE (p52)

BOTTOM
Ground through
your sitting bones
to lengthen your
spine away from
your waist

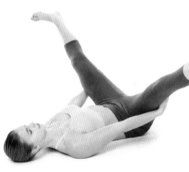

⑤ RECLINING WIDE ANGLE POSE (p85)

THIGHS
Allow the weight of
your legs to gently
open your hips

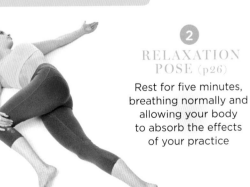

COOL DOWN/RELAXATION

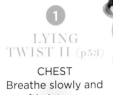

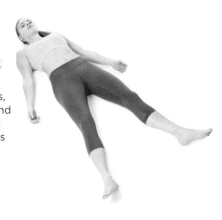

① LYING TWIST II (p53)

CHEST
Breathe slowly and
softly into your
lower belly, side ribs
and upper chest

② RELAXATION POSE (p26)

Rest for five minutes,
breathing normally and
allowing your body
to absorb the effects
of your practice

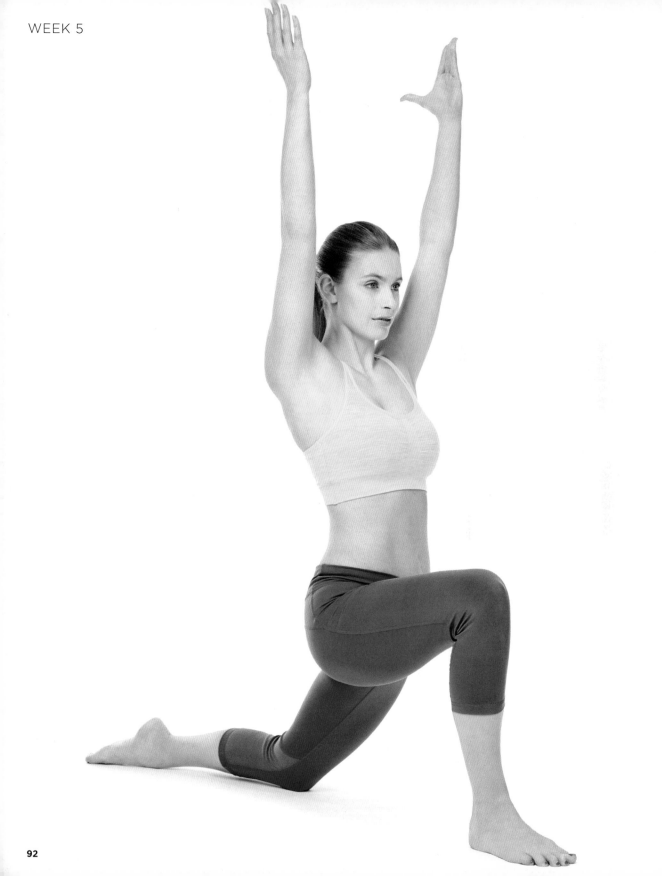

Week 5

One of the joys of yoga is that it brings mental as well as physical benefits. This week will be a **gentle and mindful** introduction to backbends, integrating what you've learnt about your pelvis and spine over the previous two weeks. Not only do backbends aid **deeper breathing** – meaning your blood is better able to nourish every cell in your body – they also encourage you to have an open heart. This can bring you greater **happiness in life**, and teach you how to be kinder to yourself as well as others.

" I will not die an unlived life.

I will not live In fear of falling or catching fire.

I choose to inhabit my days,

To allow my living to open me,

To make me less afraid,

More accessible;

To loosen my heart until it becomes a wing,

A torch, a promise.

I choose to risk my insignificance,

To live so that which came to me as seed

And that which came to me as blossom,

Goes on as fruit "

I will not die an unlived life
by Dawna Markova
Inspirational speaker and writer

THIS WEEK'S FOCUS

GENTLE BACKBENDS

Yoga isn't just about physical benefits – calmness, inner strength and confidence can also be reached. And poses can help create a specific outcome – forward bends are calming, while backbends can energise

This week, we'll be integrating the poem on page 95 into your practice, to set the scene for deeper self-reflection. Stress, past hurts and the busy pace of modern life can leave us out of touch with our feelings, who we truly are and, therefore, our present and future needs – physical, emotional and spiritual. Working gently and mindfully with backbends not only enhances spinal mobility and disc health, it also helps us open to ourselves and others.

There are several things you can do to take care of yourself as you work with backbends. It's important to stay grounded, so direct your attention to the part of your body that is in contact with the ground, and imagine directing your out-breath down your body and into the floor. Use pada and hasta bandha, and begin to become familiar with lengthening your spine away from your waist. A good way to practise this is to place your hands on your hips and, as you inhale, draw your spine upwards, crown of your head to the ceiling. Release on an exhale then repeat. Once you're familiar with this feeling, you can try using the technique in your postures. This week we'll also work on mobilising the shoulder joint and increasing your core awareness to help support your lower back.

Your Week 5 yoga sessions

Create a gentle, nurturing place to practise this week. You might like to light a candle, have some fragrant flowers near your mat or air the room before you begin. Start by spending a few moments in Easy (p24) or Accomplished (p25) poses to soften your breath and quieten your mind, then check in with how you are feeling before moving into your practice. If you're designing your own sessions, remember to warm your body up well and always include a twist before you go into backbends.

(p24) (p25)

SUGGESTED PLAN

Session 1 (25 minutes) Relaxation pose with chest opener, 2 warm-up poses, Beginner's sun salute plus Full crescent, Prayer twist and sitting poses

Session 2 (25 minutes) 2 warm-up poses, Beginner's sun salute plus Full crescent and standing poses, including Warrior flow

Session 3 (1 hour) Week 5 sequence

WEEK FIVE

NEW POSES

✦ Relaxation pose with chest opener

✦ Full crescent

✦ Boat

✦ Locust

✦ Plough

NEW SEQUENCE

✦ Warrior flow

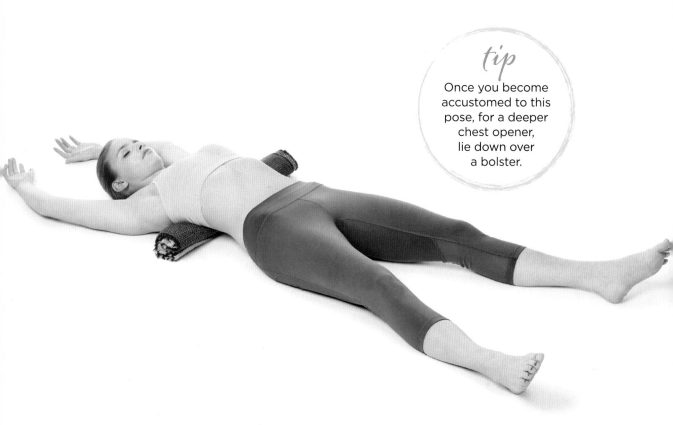

tip

Once you become accustomed to this pose, for a deeper chest opener, lie down over a bolster.

RELAXATION POSE WITH CHEST OPENER
Savasana with chest opener

● Before you lie down, place a rolled up blanket horizontally across your mat, about a third of the way from the top.
● Lie down on your back, adjusting the position of the blanket if needed, so that it supports your upper ribs, around the height of your bra. Take your arms out to the sides or overhead, whichever feels most comfortable for you, palms facing upwards, and separate your legs a little wider than hip-distance apart, allowing your ankles to naturally fall out to the sides. Rest on the centre of the back of your head, and lengthen the back of your neck.
● Mentally scan your body to ensure that your limbs are symmetrical and your legs are equidistant from an imaginary mid-line, then gently close your eyes.
● Spend up to five minutes breathing slowly and mindfully in the pose, releasing any tension on the out-breath. As you allow your body to mould itself around the rolled blanket, feel the expansion in your upper chest and allow your breath to naturally deepen.
● When you're ready to come out of the pose, gently stretch from your fingertips to your toes, bring your knees to your chest and gently roll over to your right side before using your hands to help you come up to sitting.

GOOD FOR
✦ Deeply relaxing
✦ Opening your chest
✦ Aiding deeper breathing
✦ Calming your mind

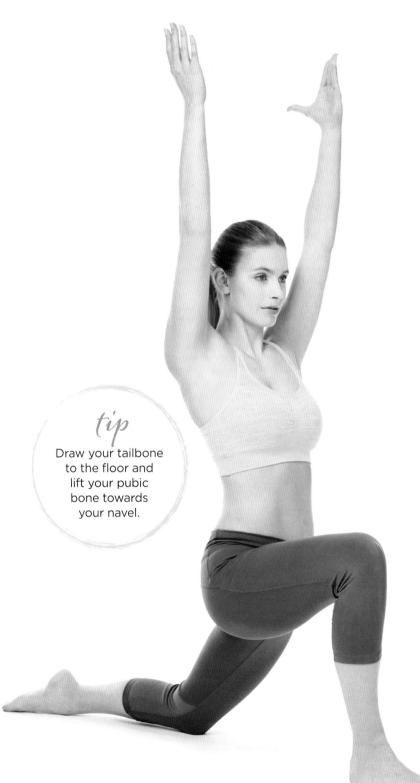

FULL CRESCENT
Anjaneyasana

- Stand with your feet shoulder-width apart, inhale then, as you exhale, fold forwards from your waist. Bend your knees as deeply as you need to bring your fingertips to the floor, one either side of your feet.
- Inhale and slide your left leg back, lowering your left knee and the top of your left foot onto the floor. Exhale. Spread the toes of your right foot, pressing down through your big and little toes. Draw your ankle out to the side to lift your inner arch.
- Square your hips to the front of the mat and breath deeply here for a few moments, then inhale and bring both hands to rest on your right knee.
- Draw your belly button towards your spine to support your lower back, square your hips to the front of the mat and release your shoulder blades down your back.
- On your next inhale, draw your belly button towards your spine to support your lower back and take your arms out to the sides and overhead, hands shoulder-width apart and palms facing.
- Take five breaths into your belly, lower on an exhale and repeat on the other side.

tip
Draw your tailbone to the floor and lift your pubic bone towards your navel.

GOOD FOR
✦ Balancing your nervous system
✦ Energising without overstimulating
✦ Helpful for sciatica

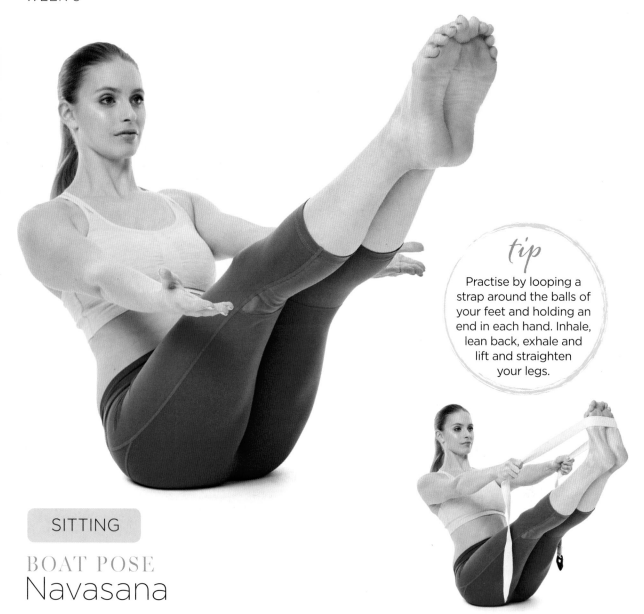

tip

Practise by looping a strap around the balls of your feet and holding an end in each hand. Inhale, lean back, exhale and lift and straighten your legs.

SITTING

BOAT POSE
Navasana

● Sit on your mat, bend your knees, raise your feet off the floor and grasp the back of your thighs with your hands.

● Draw your navel to your spine and lean back to balance on your sitting bones. Take a few breaths here, then raise your lower legs until your thighs are at 45 degrees and your shins are parallel to the floor. Draw your shoulder blades down your spine and keep your abdominals engaged, but your feet relaxed.

● Lengthen your tailbone into the floor and lift your pubis towards your navel. If you are comfortable here, extend your arms and hold them parallel to the floor, extending right through to your fingertips. Take another few breaths, and, if you feel balanced, straighten your legs to take your body into a 'V' shape.

● Tuck your chin in slightly so that the base of your skull lifts lightly away from the back of your neck. Take up to five breaths, before releasing on an exhale.

GOOD FOR
✦ Aiding focus
✦ Easing stress
✦ Toning your abdominals
✦ Strengthening your back muscles

LOCUST
Salabasana

● Lie on your tummy, chin resting on the mat and arms at your sides, palms facing upwards.

● Turn your big toes towards each other to rotate your thighs inwards and take a few breaths to centre yourself.

● On an inhale, draw your navel to your spine and lift your legs, extending right through to your pointed toes. At the same time, raise your head, chest and arms so that you're resting on your lower ribs, stomach and lower abdomen. Extend your arms all the way to your fingertips, imagining you're lifting them up against a weight and bring your shoulder blades in towards your back.

● Engage your glutes and reach strongly through your legs, keeping your big toes turning inwards.

● Lengthen the back of your neck and gaze gently forwards.

● Take five deep breaths, then release on an exhale.

● Rest your head on your folded arms, face pointing to the side. Then repeat two to three times more.

GOOD FOR

✦ Relieving stress
✦ Energising
✦ Opening your chest and shoulders
✦ Strengthening your legs

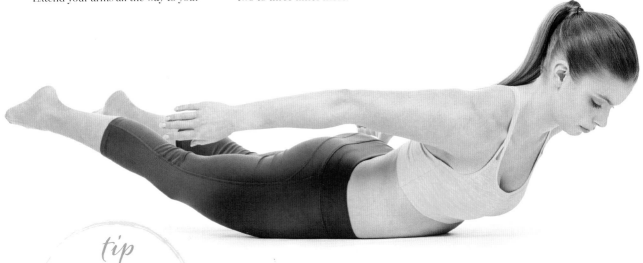

tip

If helpful, place one rolled-up blanket beneath your ribs and another beneath your front thighs to help maintain the lift.

SITTING

SUPPORTED PLOUGH

Halasana

- Lie on your back with your arms by your sides, palms down. As you exhale, push your hands into the mat, draw your navel to your spine to contract your abdominals and bring your knees to your chest, curling your body into a loose ball.
- Using this momentum, swing your feet over your head as you take your hands to your hips to support your lower back. Continue rolling back, allowing your toes to rest on the floor behind you.
- For now, slightly round your torso and keep your knees bent. Keep your gaze towards your thighs, as this will protect your neck from any damage.

- As you become acclimatised to the pose, lift your hips to bring them directly above your shoulders, draw your hands down your spine to support your upper back and begin to extend your heels away to gradually straighten your legs.
- If you feel comfortable here, clasp your hands together beneath your back, wriggle your shoulders together, and press your arms into the mat.
- Take five to 10 slow breaths, then exhale to release, bending your knees and rolling down slowly, one vertebra at a time.

tip

Practise by lowering your legs against a wall. As you build up flexibility, gradually reduce the height of the support until your feet reach the floor.

GOOD FOR

✦ Soothing your nerves

✦ Reducing hypertension

✦ Relieving palpitations

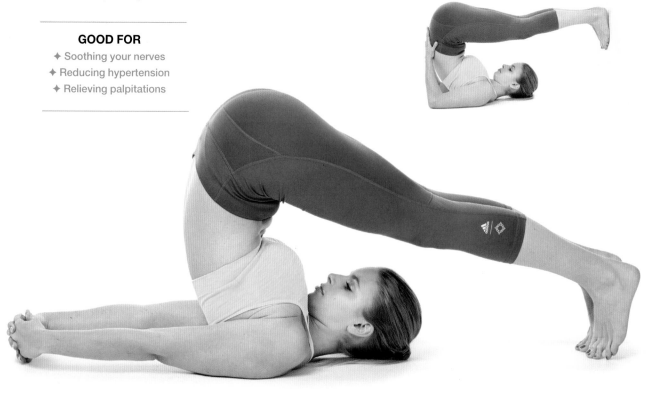

MINI SEQUENCE
Warrior flow

This sequence is an introduction to a type of yoga called vinyasa, where one pose moves straight into the next in a smooth uninterrupted flow. It's a lovely way to make yoga feel like a moving meditation, rather than a group of separate poses done one after the other

● Breathe slowly and deeply into your belly, feeling free to adjust the poses according to how you feel on the day. For example, you may want to take your hand to the floor in Extended side angle one day, but rest it on your knee another. Or try resting your back hand on your belly for Reverse warrior or your front hand on your belly for Extended side angle.

● For the first round, pause for five breaths in each pose. This will allow you to fine tune your alignment and find stillness in the flow. Repeat the sequence once or twice more, following the breathing sequence below, then swap sides.

THE FLOW
1 Warrior II (p46)
Inhale and take your front arm overhead as you slide your back arm down your leg to come into...

2 Reverse warrior (p46)
Exhale and take your front arm to your knee/the floor and circle your back arm overhead to come into...

3 Extended side angle (p48)
Inhale, engage your core, and circle your top arm back and lower arm up to shoulder height to come back into...

4 Warrior II (p46)

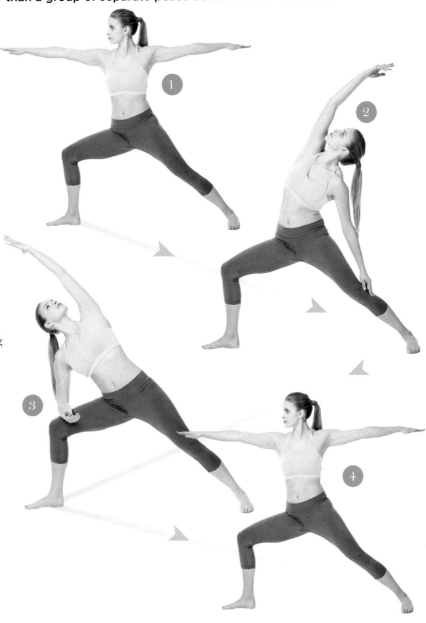

THE SEQUENCE

This week is a gentle introduction to heart-opening backbends.
We also work with twists, which prepare your spine for extension

Time: 60 minutes

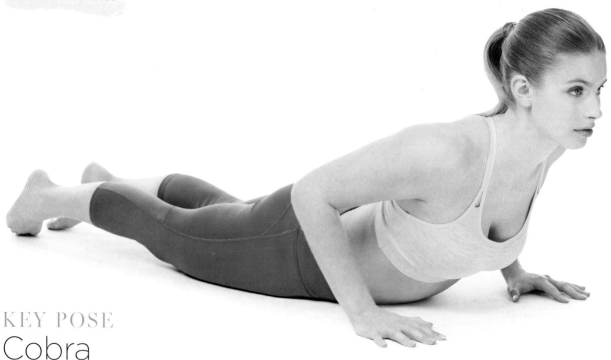

KEY POSE
Cobra

● Cobra is a classic yoga backbend. There are three possible hand positions for cobra – chosen when you are lying on the floor on your stomach. A good place to begin is with your hands next to your ribs, fingertips in line with the tops of your shoulders, but if you prefer, an easier placement is hands further forwards, so your forearms are flat on the floor. As you progress, you can take your hands to your lower ribs. Another good tip is to ensure you protect your neck.

● People often tilt their head and neck backwards to come into the pose, but it's better to keep your chin tucked into your chest initially and lift from the back of

your neck. Once you've come up fully, raise your head to look forwards. When you begin, inhale up into cobra and exhale to come down two or three times, then inhale back into the pose, take three to five deep breaths and lower on an exhale.

tip Because you're opening and expanding your heart area when you work with backbends, it can sometimes make you feel emotionally sensitive. Always trust your instincts and only go as far as feels right. If you feel uncomfortable, focus on your feet and feel them rooting into the ground. You can pause and sit for a while or do some grounding standing postures, such as Mountain pose (p29) or Warrior II (p46).

ARRIVE/PREPARE

TAKE FIVE BREATHS IN EACH POSE UNLESS OTHERWISE STATED

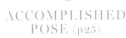

① ACCOMPLISHED POSE (p25)

Spend a few moments breathing into your belly to quieten your mind, then read the poem on page 94

② RELAXATION POSE WITH CHEST OPENER (p96)

HEART
Visualise a lotus bud in the centre of your chest, gently allowing it to open as much as feels right for you. Do this for 2 minutes

Note ....
Throughout this class, practise slow, mindful breathing to softly open your chest area

WARM-UP

① HERO TWIST (p63)

CHEST
Inhale to lengthen your spine, twist on the exhale

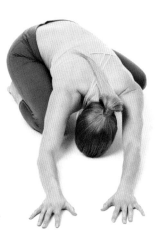

② EXTENDED CHILD'S POSE WITH SIDE STRETCH (p28)

SIDE RIBS
Breath into your side body

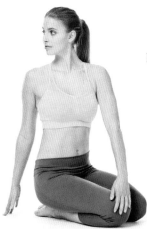

Move with your breath

Roll your shoulders back and down your spine

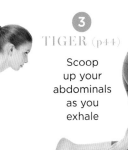

③ TIGER (p44)

Scoop up your abdominals as you exhale

103

STANDING

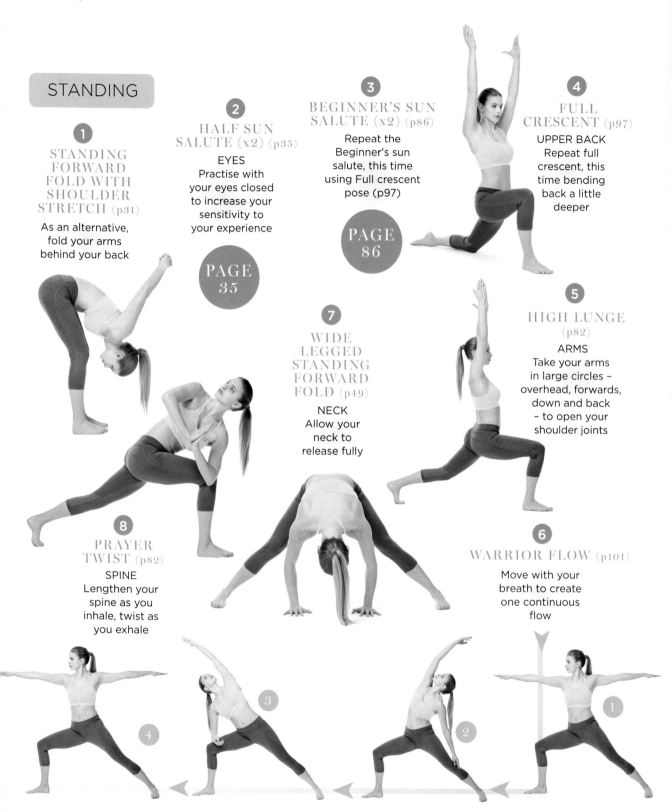

1
STANDING FORWARD FOLD WITH SHOULDER STRETCH (p31)

As an alternative, fold your arms behind your back

2
HALF SUN SALUTE (x2) (p35)

EYES
Practise with your eyes closed to increase your sensitivity to your experience

PAGE 35

3
BEGINNER'S SUN SALUTE (x2) (p86)

Repeat the Beginner's sun salute, this time using Full crescent pose (p97)

PAGE 86

4
FULL CRESCENT (p97)

UPPER BACK
Repeat full crescent, this time bending back a little deeper

5
HIGH LUNGE (p82)

ARMS
Take your arms in large circles – overhead, forwards, down and back – to open your shoulder joints

6
WARRIOR FLOW (p101)

Move with your breath to create one continuous flow

7
WIDE LEGGED STANDING FORWARD FOLD (p49)

NECK
Allow your neck to release fully

8
PRAYER TWIST (p82)

SPINE
Lengthen your spine as you inhale, twist as you exhale

SITTING

1

CAMEL (p84)

HANDS
Root through
your hands
to help lift
your chest

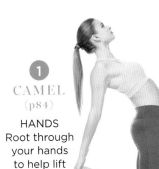

2

ACCOMPLISHED
TWIST (p25)
BACK
Draw your kidneys in
towards your back
as you twist

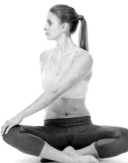

3

COBRA (p66)

Root through
your legs, pelvis
and hands
to create an
even curve in
your spine

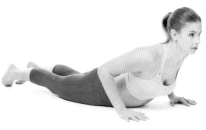

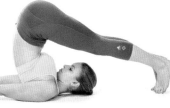

4

LOCUST (p99)

Draw your
shoulders down
your spine
to softly open
your chest

6

PLOUGH (p100)

Work towards
bringing your hips
directly over your
shoulders

5

RECLINING WIDE
ANGLE POSE (p85)

BACK
Let your back
release into the
floor completely

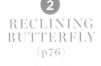

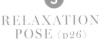

COOL DOWN/RELAXATION

1

LYING
TWIST I (p34)

Aim to keep
both shoulders
on the floor

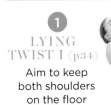

2

RECLINING
BUTTERFLY
(p76)

CHEST
Breathe softly
into your
heart area

3

RELAXATION
POSE (p26)

HEART
Visualise a soft golden
light in your heart area,
then rest one hand on
your belly and one
on your heart

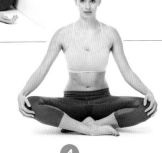

4

ACCOMPLISHED POSE (p25)

Reread the last four lines of the
poem you read at the beginning
of the session. Pause for a few
moments then circle your arms
out to the side and overhead as
you breathe in. As you exhale,
draw your hands down to prayer
position at your heart, and lower
your head for a moment or two

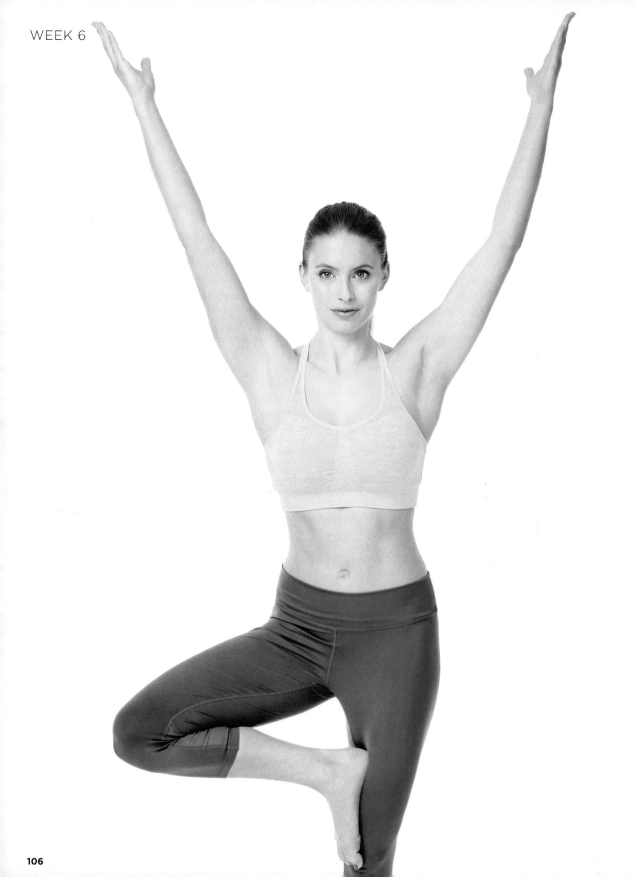

Week 6

Life is a balancing act, and your time on your mat can help prepare you for life's ups and downs. In this, the **last session** of your six-week introduction, you'll explore balancing on your feet, sitting bones and shoulders, and discover the possibility of finding equilibrium, **strength and stillness** at your centre. We finish this session with a full sun salute, balancing sequence and an invitation to open to the possibility of greater self-acceptance, no matter what is happening in your life.

" You do not have to be good.
You do not have to walk on your knees
For a hundred miles through the desert,
repenting.

You only have to let the soft animal of your body
love what it loves.

Tell me about your despair, yours,
and I will tell you mine.

Meanwhile the world goes on.

Meanwhile the sun and the clear pebbles of the rain
are moving across the landscapes, over the prairies
and the deep trees, the mountains and the rivers.

Meanwhile the wild geese, high in the clean blue air,
are heading home again.

Whoever you are, no matter how lonely,
the world offers itself to your imagination,
calls to you like the wild geese, harsh and exciting
over and over announcing your place
in the family of things "

Wild Geese
by Mary Oliver
Poet

BALANCES

Mastering balances helps you feel a sense of equilibrium and strength at your centre. Over time, you'll find it supports physical balance in your daily life, while increasing mental focus and emotional strength

There are several ways to help you feel stable in yoga balances. Ground through your feet in standing poses, such as Swaying palm tree (p114), Tree (p115) and Extended hand-to-toe pose (p116), while focusing on a point at eye level a few feet in front of you and breathing slowly and deeply into your abdomen – all techniques that, incidentally, help to keep you emotionally stable and mentally focused too. In Boat pose (p98), engaging your core and drawing your shoulders down your spine will help to stabilise your torso and, in Shoulder stand (p118), root down with your forearms while using your core to lift your torso and legs.

Finally, let your balance poses be alive. Even the strongest trees sway in the wind – their ability to adapt and respond to external forces is one of the ways they enhance their chance of survival. In your Tree posture, as well as in other balances, the tiny stablising muscles in your body will be constantly adapting to keep you balanced. Rather than forcefully contracting your body in an attempt to stay balanced or being too relaxed to maintain a posture for more than a few seconds, be flexible in your approach until you find the middle position – poised between the two extremes.

Your Week 6 yoga sessions

In your practice this week, whenever you want to feel more balanced in your life, practise a few rounds of Nadi shodana (p111). To help you work on the balance poses, once you've become familiar with Reclining tree (p113), practise the standing version at home when you have a spare few minutes. Simply rest one hand on a free wall and spend a couple of moments grounding through your supporting foot as you raise your opposite leg to your ankle, calf or higher. It's a great way to take the fear out of balance poses.

WEEK SIX

NEW POSES
+ Nadi shodana
+ Reclining hand-to-toe II
+ Reclining tree
+ Swaying palm tree
+ Tree
+ Extended hand-to-toe II
+ Lord of the fishes
+ Shoulder stand

NEW SEQUENCE
+ Classic sun salute

SUGGESTED PLAN

Session 1 (30 minutes) Reclining tree and Reclining head-to-toe pose, Classic sun salute and standing poses

Session 2 (30 minutes) Tiger (p44), Hero (p63), Classic sun salute and seated poses

Session 3 (1 hour) Week 6 sequence

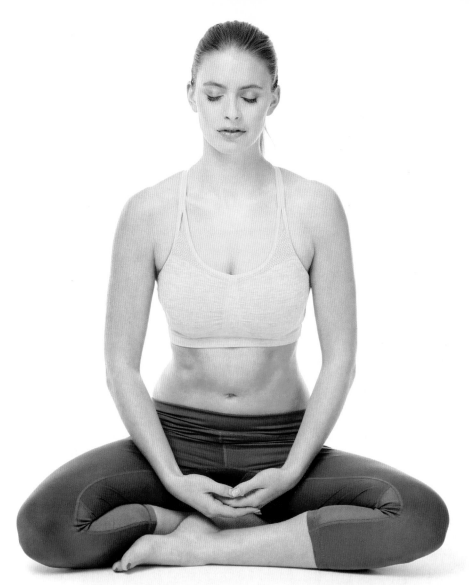

Introduction to
PRANAYAMA

At the beginning of this yoga course we introduced you to yogic breathing with the full abdominal breath (p36). This week, we'll take it a bit further with a specific breathing exercise. But first, it can be helpful to understand something of the background to the breathing practices in yoga.

● In yogic philosophy, breath is linked with prana – the energy that sustains all living things. Prana also refers to the upward movement of energy in the body, created by the in-breath. If you take a deep inhalation now, you'll soon feel fresher and lighter. Apana, the opposite of prana, is associated with the downward movement of energy and the out-breath. You can feel this for yourself when you take a long slow exhalation – notice how it makes you feel calmer, more relaxed and as if your energy is sinking downwards.

● Pranayama – yogic practices that work with controlling the breath – can bring many benefits, from calming your mind, to boosting your energy, increasing your focus and harnessing your strength and determination. On the following page, we'll look at a practice that helps create balance in your body.

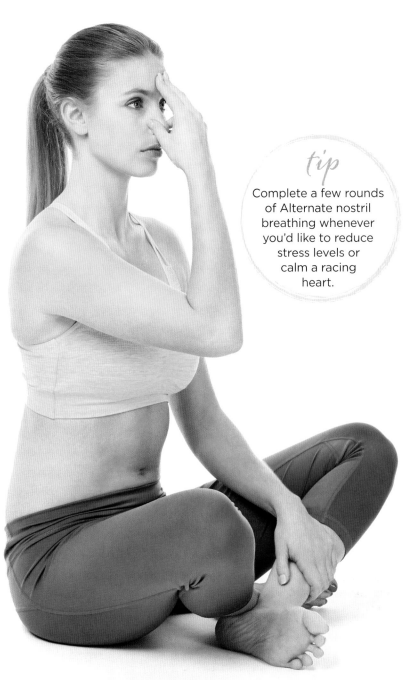

ALTERNATE NOSTRIL BREATHING
Nadi shodana

● This yogic breathing practice calms your mind and balances the right sides of your body, so is perfect to use in conjunction with balance poses.

● Sit in a comfortable position and take a moment to centre yourself. Bring your right hand to your nose, and rest the tip of your thumb on the fleshy part of your right nostril and the tips of your index and middle fingers between your eyebrows. Curl your ring and little fingers under, and rest the inside of your ring finger on your left nostril.

● Close your left nostril with your ring finger and exhale fully through your right nostril. Keeping your left nostril closed, inhale fully and slowly through your right nostril, then close your right nostril with your thumb and release your ring finger to open your left nostril and exhale slowly.

● Pause, then slowly inhale through your left nostril. Close off that nostril with your ring finger, pause, and release your right nostril with your thumb. Then exhale slowly and steadily through your right nostril.

● This forms one round. Repeat, breathing slowly and mindfully for five minutes.

tip

Complete a few rounds of Alternate nostril breathing whenever you'd like to reduce stress levels or calm a racing heart.

GOOD FOR
✦ Calming your mind
✦ Balancing the right sides of your body

RECLINING HAND-TO-TOE POSE II
Supta padangusthasana II

● Lie on your back, knees bent and feet flat on the floor, close to your buttocks. Slowly extend your right leg to lie flat on the floor, flex your ankle, spread the toes of your right foot, extending your big and little toes away from you, making sure your big toe is pointing towards the ceiling. Reach through the heel and the ball of your right foot.

● Bend your left knee in to your chest and wrap a yoga strap around the ball

of your foot, holding both ends in your left hand.

● Slowly extend your left leg upwards, taking it as close to vertical as is comfortable. Keep your ankle flexed and reach through your left heel. Inhale, then as you exhale, allow your leg to release out to the side.

● Lightly engage your core, draw your shoulders down your spine and keep both legs active. Take your right arm out

to the side, shoulder height and palm facing upwards. Take five to 10 deep breaths, walking your hands up the strap as the pose becomes more comfortable and your flexibility increases.

● When you feel ready, on an exhale, gently bring your leg back to centre and lower to the floor. Pause for a moment then repeat on the other side.

GOOD FOR
✦ Stretching your hamstrings and calves
✦ Opening your hips
✦ Relieving backache
✦ Strengthening your knees

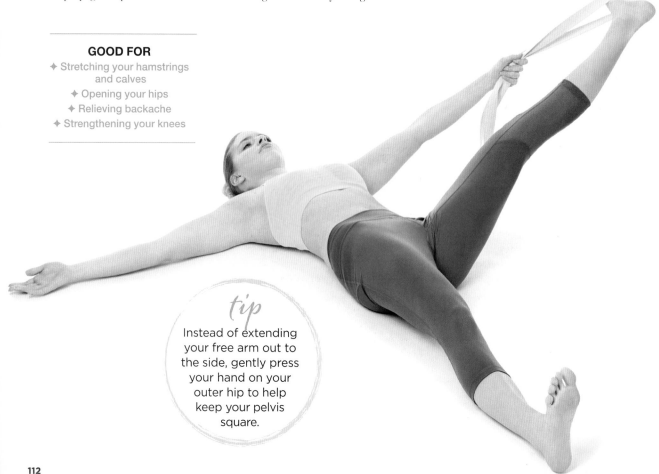

tip
Instead of extending your free arm out to the side, gently press your hand on your outer hip to help keep your pelvis square.

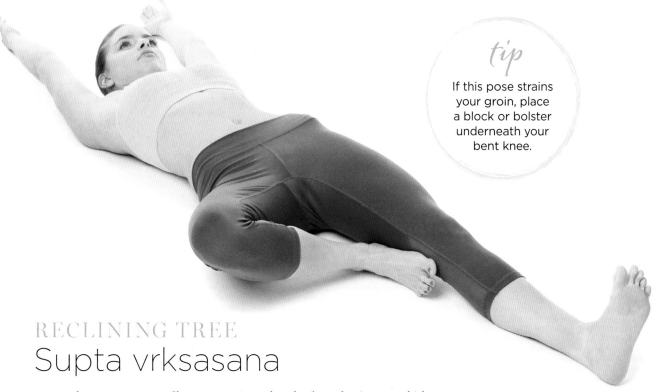

tip

If this pose strains your groin, place a block or bolster underneath your bent knee.

RECLINING TREE
Supta vrksasana

● A good way to get a sense of how tree pose should feel is to do it lying on the floor. This helps you to concentrate on the correct alignment without having to worry about your balance.

● Lie on your mat and spread the toes of your left foot, extending your big and little toes away from you, making sure your big toe is pointing towards the ceiling. Reach through the heel and ball of your foot.

● Bend your right knee and bring the sole of your right foot against the inner seam of your left calf or thigh.

Press the sole of your foot into your thigh while pressing your thigh against the sole of your foot.

● Take your right knee out to the side, keeping your hips square, and draw your navel to your spine. Keep extending through your left foot and opening your right hip. Then take your hands overhead, palms facing each other and shoulder-width apart.

● Draw your arms back into your arm sockets, take five deep breaths then exhale, and gently lower your hands and foot. Repeat on the other side.

GOOD FOR
✦ Stretching your groin, chest and shoulders
✦ Calming your mind
✦ Grounding

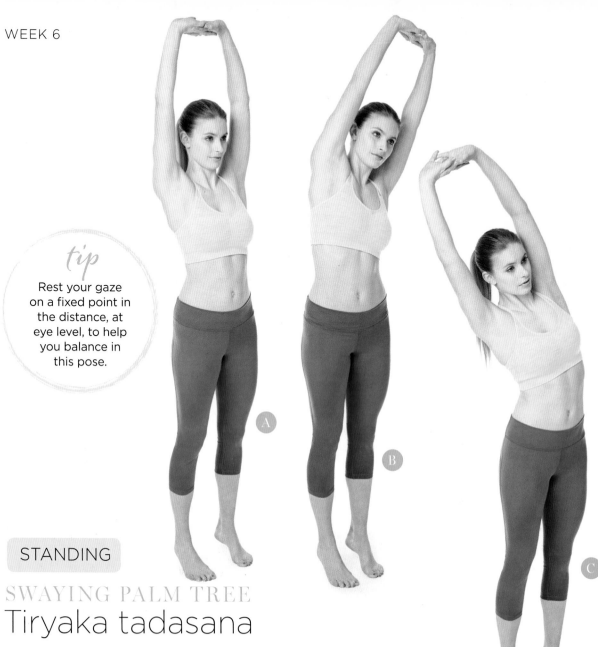

tip
Rest your gaze on a fixed point in the distance, at eye level, to help you balance in this pose.

STANDING

SWAYING PALM TREE
Tiryaka tadasana

● Stand in Mountain pose (p29), with your toes spread and rooting into the ground. Interlace your fingers, turn your palms to face away from you and take your arms overhead. On an inhale, come up on to your tip toes (A). Remain here for a couple of seconds. To help you balance, draw your leg muscles in to your bones, your navel towards your spine and your lower front ribs in slightly. Slide your shoulders down your spine to create space around your neck and gently tuck in your chin. Continue to ground through your feet to help maintain the lift, then on an exhale, gently lower your heels, and repeat once or twice more.

● On your next inhale, rise up on tip toes again and, this time, as you exhale, take your arms over to the left (B), taking care not to lean forwards as you do so. Inhale here and feel your right side opening and expanding. Exhale, then inhale as you return to the centre and repeat on the other side (C). Lower your heels on an exhale and repeat once or twice more.

GOOD FOR
✦ Grounding
✦ Aiding balance
✦ Stretching your side body
✦ Aiding deeper breathing

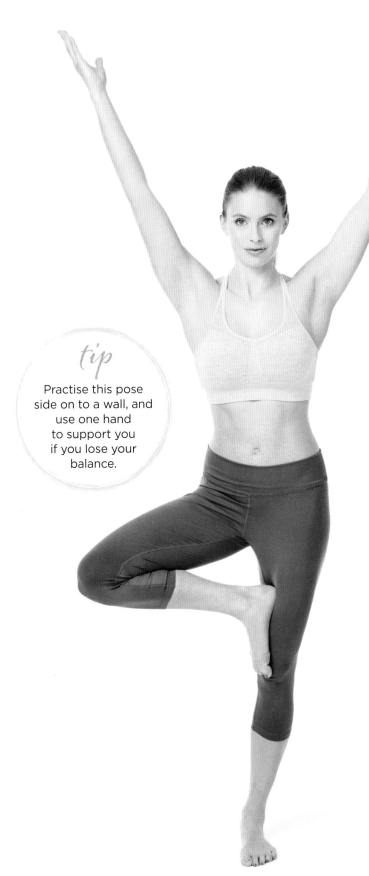

STANDING

TREE
Vrksasana

● From standing, transfer your weight onto your left leg. Spread your toes and ground through the base of your big and little toes. Lift your inner arch.

● Maintain a micro-bend in your left knee and place the sole of your right foot against the inner seam of your left calf or thigh. You can use your hand to help you place your foot if that is easier. Avoid placing your foot against your knee as this could damage the joint.

● Rest your hands on your hips while you establish your balance – pressing the sole of your foot into your thigh while pressing your thigh against the sole of your foot will help stabilise you, as will focusing on a point straight ahead of you.

● Draw your right knee out to the side, your tailbone towards the floor and your belly to your spine. Root down as you lift out of your waist and up through your crown. Bring your hands to prayer position at your heart then, if you feel well balanced, slowly glide your hands overhead.

● Take five deep breaths then exhale, gently lower your hands and foot, and repeat on the other side.

GOOD FOR
✦ Mental and physical balance
✦ Stretching your groin, chest and shoulders
✦ Calming your mind
✦ Grounding

STANDING

EXTENDED HAND-TO-TOE POSE II
Utthita hasta padangusthasana II

● From standing, transfer your weight over your left foot. Spread your toes and ground yourself through the base of your big and little toes. Lift your inner arch.
● Raise your right knee to hip height and clasp it with your right hand. Continue to root through your left foot as you extend your left arm out to the side. Take three to five breaths. Release on an exhale, then repeat on the other side.
● Next, stand by a wall and wrap a strap around the ball of your right foot, holding the ends in your right hand. Rest your left hand against the wall.
● Draw your navel to your spine, your shoulders down your back and lift though the crown. When you feel ready, exhale and extend your right leg out to the side, using the strap as support and directing your energy out through your extended limbs. Your leg may be bent initially, but over time, you'll be able to straighten it as your balance improves.
● To come out of the pose, exhale and gently lower your hands and foot. Pause for a moment before repeating on the other side.

GOOD FOR
✦ Balance
✦ Strength
✦ Steadiness
✦ Focus

tip
Gradually shorten the length of the strap as you gain flexibility and strength. Once you feel confident, remove the strap and come away from the wall.

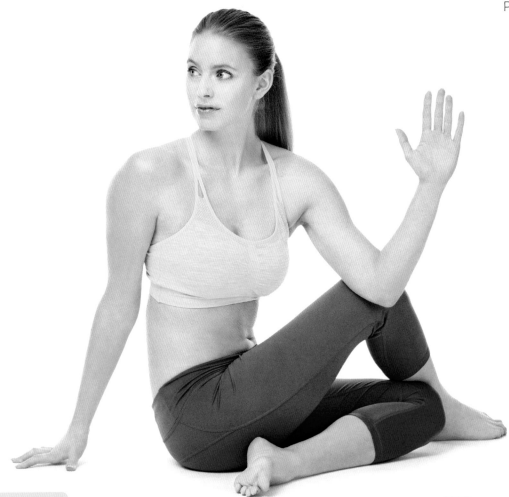

SITTING

LORD OF THE FISHES
Ardha matsyendrasana

● From Staff pose (p50), place your right foot outside your left knee, toes forwards and right knee pointing to the ceiling. Bend your left knee and slide your left foot to the outside of your right hip. Root down through your sitting bones.

● Wrap your left arm around your right knee and rest your right fingertips on the floor behind you. If comfortable, inhale to raise your left hand, and on an exhale, take your elbow outside your right knee, forearm vertical and palm facing the right. Keep your spine

vertical and draw your shoulder blades into your back.

● Inhale as you root through your fingers and sitting bones to lengthen your spine, then as you exhale, twist to the right. Move a little deeper into the stretch with each breath, lengthening your spine on the inhale, releasing a little deeper into the twist on the exhale.

● Turn your head to gaze over your right shoulder, breathing evenly from your belly for another five breaths. Inhale to come back to the centre, then pause before repeating on the other side.

tip

If one sitting bone comes off of the floor, or your back rounds, place a folded blanket or block underneath it.

GOOD FOR

✦ Easing tension in your back
✦ Toning your spinal nerves
✦ Opening your chest
✦ Relieving stiff hips

117

SITTING

SUPPORTED SHOULDER STAND
Salamba sarvangasana

Known as the queen of yoga poses, practising shoulder stand regularly is believed to balance the nervous and endocrine systems. Because it's such an important asana, it's worth taking time to learn the pose in detail

● Good preparatory poses include anything that opens your shoulders, such as Hero with cow face arms (p79) or Standing forward fold with shoulder stretch (p81). So if you practise Shoulder stand on its own, it can be very helpful to start with these.

● When you first begin to work with Supported shoulder stand it's a good idea to use blankets to support your neck. Your cervical spine is very vulnerable in this pose as your head is bent at such an extreme angle, so until you learn to take the weight of your body completely on your head, shoulders and the backs of your arms, some padding can be useful.

● Fold two or more firm blankets into a rectangle measuring about 30cm by 60cm and place them on your mat, one on top of the other. The long side of the rectangle should be parallel to the short end of your mat.

● To come into the pose, lie on your back and position yourself so that your head is on the floor and your shoulders are on the blankets. Have about 5cm between the tops of your shoulders and the edge of the blanket. Bend your knees and place your feet on the floor, heels close to your sitting bones and arms by your sides, palms facing downwards.

● Engage your core and, on an exhale, push your feet into the floor to roll onto your upper back, lifting your legs to take your hips over your shoulders. Bring your hands to your hips, to support your lower back. Keep your legs bent initially, with your thighs parallel to the ground and your calves at 45 degrees (A). Rest here for a moment or two until you become acclimatised to the pose.

● When you feel ready, tuck your shoulders under and bring your elbows closer together, so they're about shoulder-width apart and walk your hands down your back (closer to the floor). Gradually straighten your legs, taking them to a 45-degree angle to the floor (B).

● If you feel comfortable here, engage your abdomen and lift your legs to vertical, keeping your leg muscles strong and your toes reaching towards the ceiling (C). Aim to hover your toes over your shoulders rather than over your head.

● Keep drawing your abdomen towards your spine, your upper back towards your chest and lift the sides of your body and pelvis towards the ceiling. Lift your buttocks away from your lower back until your torso is perpendicular to the floor and continue lifting through your legs. To keep your neck safe, keep your chin pointing up towards the ceiling.

● Take up to 20 deep breaths, then to come down, bend your knees, round your back and roll down slowly onto the mat, using your hands to support your back as you do so.

GOOD FOR

✦ Soothing stress

✦ Easing tiredness

✦ Stretching your shoulders and back

✦ Stimulating your thyroid gland

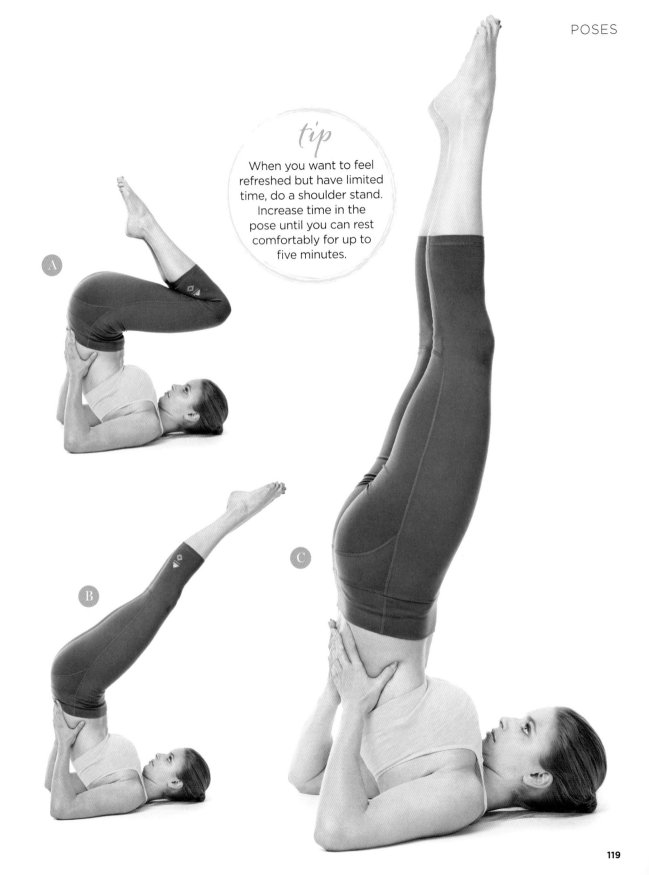

tip

When you want to feel refreshed but have limited time, do a shoulder stand. Increase time in the pose until you can rest comfortably for up to five minutes.

A

B

C

MINI SEQUENCE
Classic sun salute

Now that you've learnt all the poses in a Classic sun salute, it's time to give the full sequence a try

● Move slowly and mindfully, listening to your body and following what it needs. On the first round, if it feels appropriate, explore using free movement in Crescent (p80), Downward dog (p65) and Cobra (p66), moving your spine, shoulders, arms and neck in a slow fluid way to bring more freedom to your body. For example, releasing your arms and twisting your spine in Crescent, or swaying your hips from side to side as you bend alternate knees. This will help you let go of any unnecessary tension and arrive more fully in the present moment.

● As with the Beginner's sun salute (p86), take five breaths in each pose on the first round, then follow the breathing pattern below for subsequent rounds. Use your breath to expand your body fully as you inhale, release and soften as you exhale.

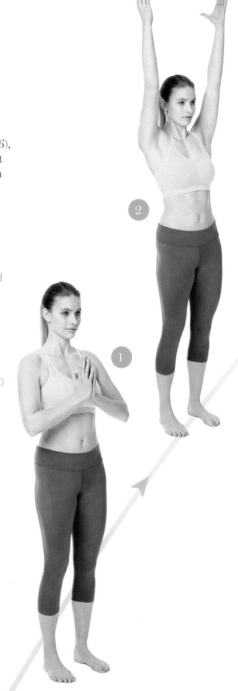

1 Mountain pose prayer hands (p29)
Inhale, root through your feet and take your arms out to the sides and overhead to...

2 Extended mountain pose (p30)
Exhale and take your arms to the sides and down into...

3 Standing forward fold (p31)
Inhale as you step your left leg back to...

4 Full crescent (p80)
Exhale and step your right foot back to...

5 Downward dog (p65)
Take five deep breaths here, 'walking the dog' by bending one knee then the other, and focus on lifting your tailbone up and back to lengthen your spine.

6 Caterpillar
Pause the breath as you lower your knees and chest to the floor, and then your abdomen. Then inhale into...

7 Cobra (p66)
Exhale and root through your hands to lift back into...

8 Downward dog (p65)
Inhale as you step your left foot forward into...

9 Full crescent (p80)
Exhale and step your right foot into...

10 Standing forward fold (p31)
Inhale, taking your arms out to the side and overhead to...

11 Extended mountain pose (p30)
Exhale your arms out to the side and to prayer, back into...

12 Mountain pose (p29)
Repeat, leading with your right leg. This forms one round.

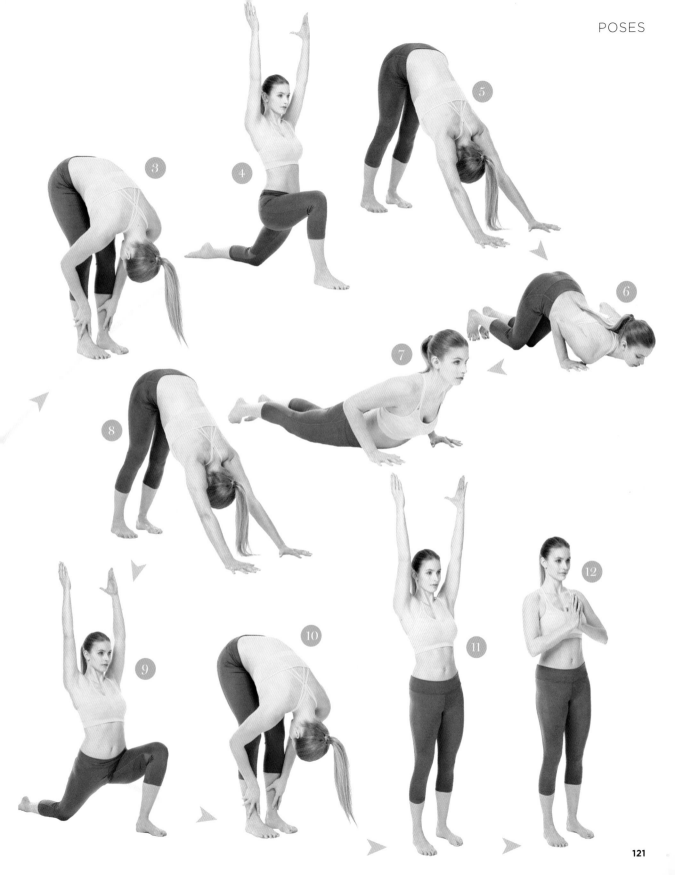

THE SEQUENCE

This week is a gentle introduction to heart-opening backbends.
We also work with twists, which prepare the spine for extension

Time: 60 minutes

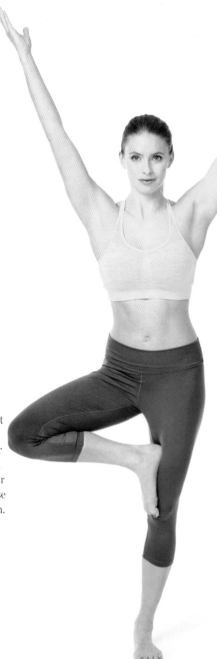

KEY POSE
Tree

● Tree pose is an iconic yoga balance and, after a little practice, once you become familiar with its key alignment points, you'll be surprised at the deep sense of calm, focus and harmony it can bring to you. A quality of presence that you'll be able to draw on when you're not on your yoga mat. Start simply, perhaps at a wall or balancing on the toes of your bent leg, heel resting against your ankle, or place the sole of your foot against your calf. As you become more confident, raise your foot to the inner seam of your thigh. Just avoid your knee as the sideways pressure could damage the joint. You could also start with your hands on your hips or in prayer position at your heart. As with all standing poses, a strong foundation, firm core and shoulder blades hugging your back will give you a sense of solidity.

tip Music can be a wonderful way to support your yoga practice. For this last class, choose one of your favourite calming tracks to help you sink more deeply into the postures. Alternatively, try *Invocation* by Ty Burhoe or anything by Deva Premal.

ARRIVE/PREPARE

TAKE FIVE BREATHS IN EACH POSE UNLESS OTHERWISE STATED

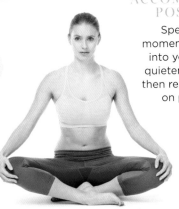

1 ACCOMPLISHED POSE (p25)

Spend a few moments breathing into your belly to quieten your mind, then read the poem on page 108

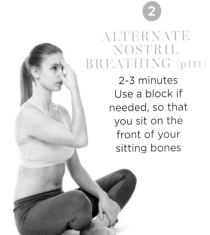

2 ALTERNATE NOSTRIL BREATHING (p111)

2-3 minutes Use a block if needed, so that you sit on the front of your sitting bones

WARM-UP

Throughout this class, to aid your balance, focus on a fixed point in front of you, at eye level

PELVIS Instigate the movement from your pelvis

2 HERO WITH COW FACE ARMS (p79)

SHOULDERS If your shoulders feel tight, direct your breath to the area to help release any tension

3 RECLINING HEAD-TO-TOE II (p112)

HIPS If needed, use your extended hand to keep your hips level

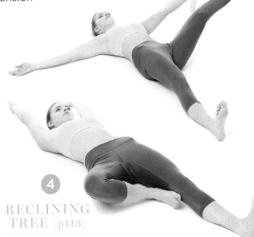

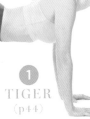

1 TIGER (p44)

NECK Let your neck release to the floor

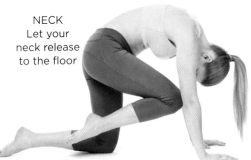

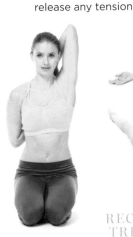

4 RECLINING TREE (p113)

WHOLE BODY Keep the pose active, even though you're lying on the floor

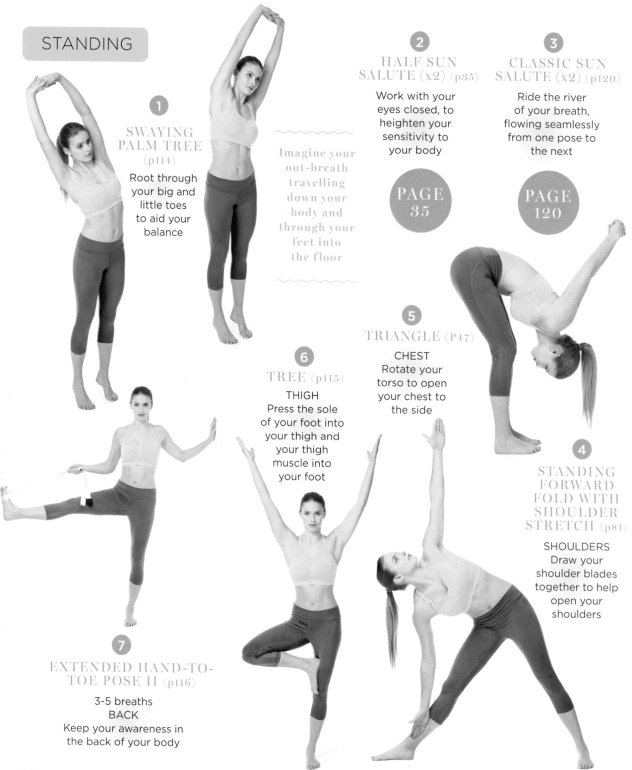

STANDING

1

SWAYING
PALM TREE
(p114)

Root through
your big and
little toes
to aid your
balance

*Imagine your
out-breath
travelling
down your
body and
through your
feet into
the floor*

2

HALF SUN
SALUTE (x2) (p35)

Work with your
eyes closed, to
heighten your
sensitivity to
your body

PAGE
35

3

CLASSIC SUN
SALUTE (x2) (p120)

Ride the river
of your breath,
flowing seamlessly
from one pose to
the next

PAGE
120

5

TRIANGLE (P47)

CHEST
Rotate your
torso to open
your chest to
the side

6

TREE (p115)

THIGH
Press the sole
of your foot into
your thigh and
your thigh
muscle into
your foot

4

STANDING
FORWARD
FOLD WITH
SHOULDER
STRETCH (p81)

SHOULDERS
Draw your
shoulder blades
together to help
open your
shoulders

7

EXTENDED HAND-TO-
TOE POSE II (p116)

3-5 breaths
BACK
Keep your awareness in
the back of your body

SITTING

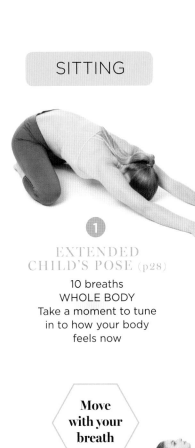

❷ LORD OF THE FISHES (p117)

ELBOW
Use your elbow to help you move deeper into the twist

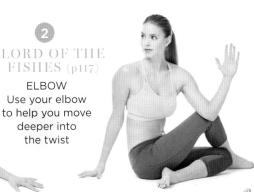

❸ BOAT POSE (p98)

TORSO
Draw your shoulders down your spine and engage your core

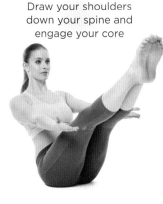

❶ EXTENDED CHILD'S POSE (p28)

10 breaths
WHOLE BODY
Take a moment to tune in to how your body feels now

❺ BRIDGE (p32)

FOOT
Reach your top foot up to the ceiling

❹ SHOULDER STAND (p118)

UPPER ARMS
Aim to keep your upper arms parallel

Move with your breath

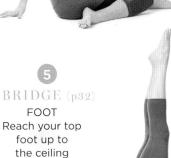

COOL DOWN/RELAXATION

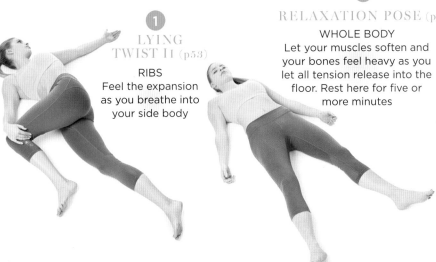

❶ LYING TWIST II (p53)

RIBS
Feel the expansion as you breathe into your side body

❷ RELAXATION POSE (p26)

WHOLE BODY
Let your muscles soften and your bones feel heavy as you let all tension release into the floor. Rest here for five or more minutes

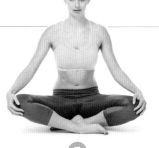

❸ ACCOMPLISHED POSE (p25)

Reread the first five lines of the poem you read at the start of your session, then pause to allow the words to sink in. Circle your arms out to the side and overhead as you breathe in. As you exhale, draw your hands to prayer position at your heart, and gently lower you head

Taking it
FURTHER

Keen to take your yoga journey to the next stage?
Use the following suggestions to delve more
deeply into the world of yoga

Congratulations! Now that you've completed your six-week introduction to yoga you'll be feeling the benefits of a regular practice – increased calm, greater strength and flexibility, plus a feeling of being more grounded and present in your everyday life. So what's next? The following advice will help you decide on the best way to take your yoga journey forwards. As always, listen to your own innate wisdom, and follow the path that most resonates with what you need.

1 Join a class
We hope that this book has given you the confidence to join a yoga class. Practising yoga with a group of people creates a beautiful atmosphere and sense of community that's uplifting in itself. Use the guide at the front of the book (p12-14) to help you decide which style you might prefer, then try out a few classes. Now that you know the basics, you may feel ready to join a beginner's class, or if you want to push yourself a little further, you could try a level one class. You could also attend a general class, where the teacher offers modifications for people of different levels. Give the class at least two sessions before deciding if it's right for you, and speak to the teacher to ask their advice and answer any questions you may have. Yoga classes vary enormously in price, from £5 in a rural town hall to £20 in a slick city studio, but however much you pay, it's important that you chose the right one for you.

2 Go online
If you can't get to a local class, streaming one into your living room is a great way to experience a wide variety of teachers. It's also a very cost-effective way to learn, with membership starting at about £10 a month for unlimited access to literally thousands of classes aimed at all levels. You can often choose the duration of the class (from 10 to 90 minutes), the teacher, the style and even the theme, such as a specific body part, stress-busting, morning or evening yoga and pregnancy. Our favourite site, ekhartyoga.com, also includes talks, meditations, chanting, mindfulness and programmes lasting from a few days to several weeks. You can usually sign up for free classes or a month's free trial to get a taste of what the sites offer before you commit to membership. See page 127 for other streaming inspiration.

3 Read more
Yoga books go into great detail on postures and give you time to learn at your own pace. You can also read more about the philosophy of yoga than there may be time to cover in class. Or

tip
Why not treat yourself to a gift to mark the end of the first stage of your yoga journey, such as a lavender-scented eyebag or a chakra bracelet?

you might prefer yoga flash cards. Use them to work on specific poses or create your own sequence – they often come with sequencing tips. Lay the cards out on the floor in front of your yoga mat as a visual reminder. See our reading recommendations on page 127 for books and cards that are ideal for the next stage of your practice.

4 Choose the right teacher
While you can learn a lot from a book, working with a yoga teacher will personalise your experience. A teacher can give you individual pointers and hands-on adjustments that will enable you to experience the pose more fully. Look for the following:

Training: It's possible to train as a yoga teacher in just one month, but a longer two-year course enables prospective teachers to go into much more depth,

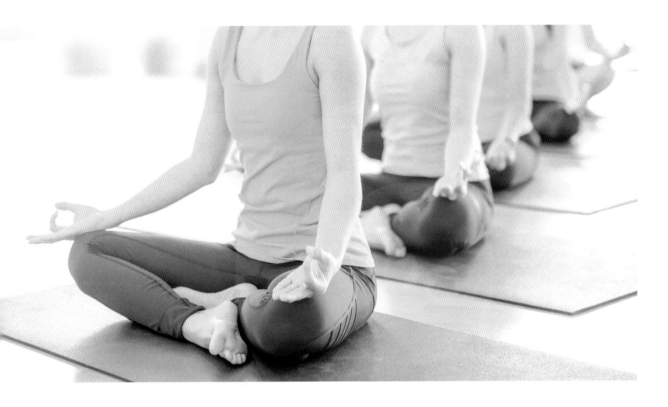

as well as to integrate what they've learnt. Read a teacher's biog on the studio's website to learn about their training and experience, or speak to them in person. The British Wheel of Yoga (bwy.org.uk) lists teachers who have completed a comprehensive BWY training. Check out its website to find an accredited teacher in your area.

Approachability: Chose someone with a friendly, open attitude, who is happy to answer any questions you have. If you resonate with your teacher this will be reflected in your practice.

Responsiblity: A good teacher should ask students about any injuries they may have at the beginning of each class and offer adjustments to prevent further damage or strain.

Commitment: Finally, a teacher committed to their own practice will be constantly learning and able to bring fresh ideas to the class.

FIND OUT MORE

Books
✦ *The Breathing Book* by Donna Farhi (Holt, £15.99)
✦ *Yoga Mind, Body & Spirit* by Donna Farhi (Gill Books, £19.99)
✦ *Yoga: The Path to Holistic Health* by BSK Iyengar (Dorling Kindersly, £25)
✦ *Yoga: The Spirit and Practice of Moving into Stillness* by Erich Schiffmann (Gallery Books, £14.99)

Yoga cards
✦ *The Mark Stephens Yoga Sequencing Deck* (North Atlantic Books, £25)

✦ *New Yoga Flash Cards* by Elisa de Dios (ISBN-10: 8461557271, £14.99)

Streaming websites
✦ ekhartyoga.com
✦ gaia.com
✦ movementformodernlife.co.uk
✦ yogaglo.com
✦ yogaia.com

Local studio finder
✦ yogafinder.com
✦ yogahub.co.uk

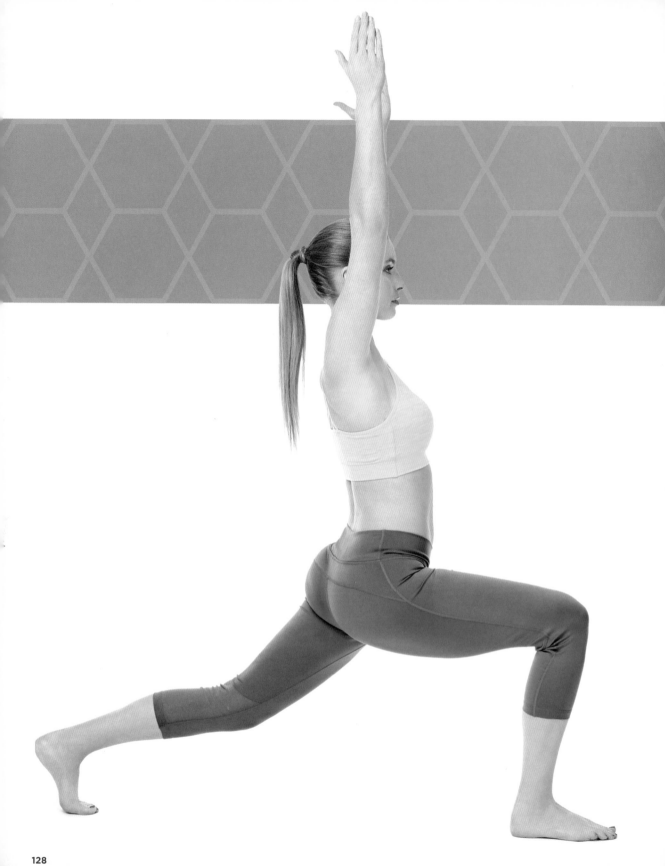

Directory

APPAREL

ACTIVE IN STYLE
activeinstyle.co.uk

ASQUITH
asquithlondon.com

EVERY SECOND COUNTS
everysecondcounts.co.uk

FROMYOGA
fromclothing.com

ILU
ilufitwear.com

LULULEMON
lululemon.co.uk

MADEBYYOGIS
yogaclicks.store

MANDUKA
manduka.com

MANUKA
manukalife.com

NOBALLS
noballs.co.uk

PURE LIME
purelimeshop.com

STYLE PB
stylepb.com

SWEATY BETTY
sweatybetty.co.uk

UNDER THE SAME SUN
underthesamesun.se

WELLICIOUS
wellicious.com

EQUIPMENT

EKOTEX YOGA
ekotexyoga.co.uk

GAIAM
gaiam.co.uk

HOLISTIC SILK
holisticsilk.com

MADEBYYOGIS
yogaclicks.store

MANDUKA
manduka.com

YOGA BLISS
yogabliss.co.uk

YOGA MATTERS
yogamatters.com

YOGA STUDIO
yogastudio.co.uk

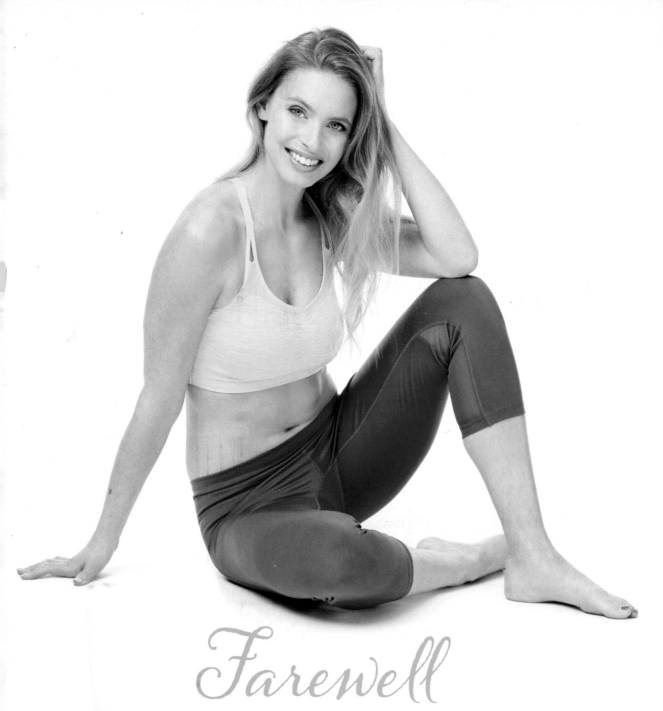

Farewell

We hope that you've enjoyed taking your first steps into the world of yoga and are reaping the benefits of a regular practice. Taking time out of your busy life to still your mind through yogic breathing, postures and meditative flows will bring a sense of peace and harmony that you can draw on whenever you need, whether you're on your mat or not! Continue to trust your body and your inner guide, and you'll find a whole new world opens up to you. We hope you enjoy your travels.